THE ASBESTOS HAZARD

THE ASBESTOS HAZARD

Paul Brodeur

The New York Academy of Sciences
New York, New York
1980

Library of Congress Cataloging in Publication Data

Brodeur, Paul.
The asbestos hazard.

Based on health hazards of asbestos exposure, the proceedings of a conference held in New York in June of 1978, by the New York Academy of Sciences, which were published as vol. 330 of the Annals of the New York Academy of Sciences.

1. Asbestosis. 2. Asbestos industry—Hygienic aspects.
3. Asbestos—Toxicology. 4. Environmentally induced diseases. I. Title.
RC775.A8B76 616.2′44 79-25221

The New York Academy of Sciences believes that it has a responsibility to encourage the dissemination of scientific information. For this reason, *The Asbestos Hazard* was written for the general public on the basis of the proceedings of an academy conference entitled Health Hazards of Asbestos Exposure. The full proceedings of the conference have been published as Volume 330 of the *Annals of the New York Academy of Sciences.* Positions taken by the conference participants whose work forms the basis for this volume are their own and not those of The Academy. The Academy has no intent to influence legislation by the publishing of such opinions.

PCP
Printed in the United States of America
ISBN 0-89766-042-0

Contents

Acknowledgments .... *vi*

PART I—INTRODUCTION 1

Chapter 1—What Is Asbestos? 4

Chapter 2—Asbestos Disease 8

Chapter 3—A History of Asbestos Disease 12

PART II—THE ORDEAL OF THE WORLD'S ASBESTOS WORKERS 17

Chapter 4—The Insulation Workers 18

Chapter 5—Miners and Millers 22

Chapter 6—The Factory Workers 29

Chapter 7—The Shipyard Problem 34

Chapter 8—Indirect Occupational Exposure 41

Chapter 9—Asbestos and Cigarettes: A Deadly Combination 44

Chapter 10—Caring for Sick Workers 46

PART III—PREVENTING OCCUPATIONAL ASBESTOS DISEASE 53

Chapter 11—Methods of Control 54

Chapter 12—How Standards Are Set 59

PART IV—THE ENVIRONMENTAL PROBLEM 65

Chapter 13—Unsuspecting Victims 67

Chapter 14—A Turkish Nightmare 73

Chapter 15—Contaminated Schools 76

Chapter 16—Future Environmental Problems 80

PART V—PUBLIC CONTROL OF ASBESTOS DISEASE 85

Chapter 17—What Should Society Be Doing? 87

Chapter 18—The Lesson of Asbestos Disease 92

Acknowledgments

The contents of this book are for the most part derived from an international conference held by The New York Academy of Sciences in June of 1978 entitled Health Hazards of Asbestos Exposure, part of a Science Week, the general title of which was The Scientific Basis for the Public Control of Environmental Health Hazards. The conference was chaired by Dr. Irving J. Selikoff of the Environmental Sciences Laboratory, Mount Sinai School of Medicine and Dr. E. Cuyler Hammond of the American Cancer Society. Various persons reviewed the original manuscript and made valuable suggestions. Chief among them were Dr. George M. Kingman, Dr. Ruth Lilis, Dr. Irving J. Selikoff, and Dr. J. Stumphius.

Financial support for the writing of this book was provided in part by the National Institute of Environmental Health Sciences.

Bill M. Boland
Executive Editor

Part I
INTRODUCTION

Asbestos has become one of the best known and most feared occupational and environmental hazards in the world. Scientists now estimate that of the millions of current and former workers who have been exposed to asbestos, 30 to 40 percent of those more heavily exposed can be expected to die of cancer. One in 5 of these workers will die of lung cancer. One in 10 will die from cancer of the gastrointestinal tract. And one in 15 will succumb to mesothelioma—an otherwise rare and fatal tumor of the membranes that surround the lungs and line the abdominal cavity.

In addition to the one million people who have worked directly with asbestos, millions of other workers have been indirectly or intermittently exposed to the mineral, particularly in the building trades and in shipyards. For example, between 1940 and 1945, some 4.5 million men and women worked around asbestos in American shipyards. The total number of workers exposed to asbestos since the beginning of World War II, including shipyard workers, is estimated to be between 8 and 11 million.

How many of these people will develop asbestos disease? No one knows for sure but there is mounting evidence to suggest that their cancer risk is significantly greater than that of the general population. Indeed, in the spring of 1978, Secretary of Health, Education & Welfare, Joseph A. Califano, Jr., announced that the government would undertake to inform former shipyard workers of this distressing situation. At the same time, Secretary Califano directed the Surgeon General of the United States to send an advisory letter to some 400,000 American physicians in order to notify them of the increased health hazards associated with asbestos exposure. He called asbestos "one of the most dangerous and insidious substances in the workplace."

But the asbestos hazard is not confined to the workplace. During the 1950s, 1960s and early 1970s, millions of unsuspecting city dwellers in the United States were exposed to asbestos as a result of living and working in the vicinity of construction sites where asbestos fireproofing materials were being sprayed on the steel girders of high-rise buildings. Fortunately, this practice was banned throughout the nation by the Environmental Protection Agency (EPA) in 1973. But since no one knows how much asbestos exposure it takes to produce cancer, no one has any idea of the risk these people may run. And since asbestos-induced cancer is not likely to appear until 20 to 40 years after first exposure, it is still too early for anyone to tell.

Moreover, the EPA's ban on asbestos-spray operations cannot by itself prevent further contamination of the ambient air with asbestos. Future demolition of buildings containing asbestos-fireproofing material is bound to release asbestos fibers into the air of our cities and towns. And recent developments such as the discovery of asbestos as a lining in 12 million hair dryers provide further indication that the asbestos hazard may be far greater than we had assumed.

Fifteen years ago, in October of 1964, The New York Academy of Sciences held an international conference entitled Biological Effects of Asbestos. Like the conference upon which this book is based, it was held in New York City. Although it was recognized at the 1964 meeting that much work remained to be done to define the true extent of the asbestos hazard, the peril of inhaling asbestos was clearly described by scientists and researchers from all over the world.

Nevertheless, thanks to lethargy and timidity on the part of government, gross irresponsibility on the part of some in industry, and unwillingness to become involved on the part of many in the medical and scientific communities, almost 8 years went by before this warning was heeded and the first rudimentary measures were taken to protect the health of the American people from asbestos. Meanwhile, hundreds of thousands of Americans, young and old, were needlessly exposed to asbestos, with results that in many instances are certain to be tragic.

This book is intended to inform workers and people in the general population about the nature of the asbestos hazard, what is known about asbestos disease, and what is being done to control it. Unfortunately, it must also stand as a grim reminder of the necessity for far swifter and more efficient public control of occupational and environmental health hazards.

Chapter 1

What Is Asbestos?

Asbestos is a broad term for a number of fibrous silicate minerals that are found in practically every country in the world. The most common variety is chrysotile, or white asbestos, which accounts for 95 percent of the world's production. The largest deposits of chrysotile are located in the Province of Quebec, in Canada, and in the Ural Mountains of the Soviet Union. In the United States, chrysotile is mined chiefly in California and Vermont.

The two other major varieties of asbestos—crocidolite and amosite—are similar to chrysotile but possess different structural and chemical properties. Crocidolite is widely known as blue asbestos, and amosite is sometimes referred to as brown asbestos. Large quantities of crocidolite and amosite are mined in South Africa. Less common varieties of asbestos include anthophyllite, tremolite, and actinolite.

Asbestos possesses some astonishing physical properties. Most people are aware that it is noncombustible and can withstand fierce heat. But asbestos is remarkable in many other ways. It appears to be extremely fragile, yet its fibers have a tensile strength equal to that of piano wire. It looks perishable, yet it is almost indestructible because it is not affected by corrosion and decay. Asbestos also resists the action of most acids, alkalies, and other chemical agents. Asbestos fibers are as heavy and dense as the rock from which they come, yet these same fibers are so soft and flexible that they can be woven into cloth as easily as fibers of cotton.

One of the most amazing things about asbestos is its fibrous structure. Indeed, the extent to which asbestos may continue to break down into smaller and smaller fibers is difficult to believe. Each asbestos fiber is actually a bundle of fibrils—tiny, needle-like particles—which are usually less than one micrometer (one thousandth of a millimeter) in length. Such fibrils are invisible to the naked eye. Thanks to the electron microscope, however, we know that there are about a million individual fibrils lying side by side in a linear inch of chrysotile asbestos. By comparison, only 630 human hairs can be aligned along the same distance!

Asbestos was known to man as early as the Stone Age, when it was used to reinforce the clay in pottery. During Greek and Roman times, it was discovered that asbestos could be woven into cloth. For this reason, the ancients at first believed that asbestos, like linen, was of vegetable origin. They also considered asbestos to be magical because of its incredible ability to resist heat and fire. Asbestos wicks were used in the sacred and inextinguishable lamps of the vestal virgins. And Roman emperors were dressed in asbestos funeral shrouds before being cremated.

During the Dark Ages, the Emperor Charlemagne is said to have awed warrior guests from a rival kingdom by throwing an asbestos tablecloth into the fire and then withdrawing it, intact and unsinged, from the flames. It is hardly surprising that in ancient times asbestos was called "the magic mineral."

How is asbestos used?

The world's first commercial asbestos mine was opened in Thetford, Quebec, 100 years ago. Since then asbestos has achieved enormous industrial importance because of its unique and varied physical properties. Between 1970 and 1975, the amount of asbestos fiber used in the United States averaged 800,000 tons a year. About two-thirds of this asbestos was used in building products, insulation, friction materials such as brake linings, and textiles. But the so-called magic mineral has many other uses. In fact, asbestos is an ingredient in several thousand different commercial products and processes. Here are some of them:

- **Asbestos cement.** The asbestos cement industry is by far the largest consumer of chrysotile asbestos in the world. Its products include shingles for roofing and siding, sheets for exterior and interior walls, insulation board, clapboard, and pipes to carry drinking water, sewage, and gas. The chrysotile fibers in asbestos cement act as tiny reinforcing rods.
- **Asbestos textiles.** Asbestos is spun and woven to make fireproof theater curtains, safety clothing, lagging cloth and other insulation wrapping, conveyor belting, pot holders, ironing board covers, draperies, rugs, lamp wicks, and fire hose. Woven asbestos friction materials are used in brake linings and clutch facings. Asbestos cloth is also used in seals and gaskets.
- **Asbestos paper.** Papers and felts made of asbestos are used for roofing, pipe covering, electrical insulation, and for lining stoves, heaters, and automobile mufflers. Asbestos paper is used for boiler jackets and radiator covers. Asbestos millboard, a heavier version of asbestos paper, is used for acoustical ceilings and for fireproof wallboard.
- **Asbestos floor tiles.** Vinyl and asphalt floor tiles contain anywhere from 30 percent to 50 percent short chrysotile fibers, which serve as filler and reinforcement material.
- **Plastics, paints, roof coatings, and caulking compounds.** Chrysotile asbestos is an ingredient in a wide variety of plastic compounds, ranging from frying pan handles to missile nose cones. Asbestos is used in plastic to increase hardness and resistance to heat and fire. Short chrysotile fibers are present as filler and reinforcement in many paints, coatings, and sealants.
- **Miscellaneous uses.** Asbestos filters have been used in gas masks and in the processing of fruit juices, wine, beer, medicines, and acids. Asbestos may also be an ingredient in asphalt paving. For many years, asbestos was widely employed in fireproof insulation sprayed on the steel girders of high-rise buildings. Recently, it has been discovered that asbestos was used to line the interiors of many hair dryers.

As a result of these multiple and miscellaneous applications, asbestos is found practically everywhere in modern society. There is not an automobile, airplane, train, ship, missile, or engine of any sort that does not contain asbestos in some form or other. And because it is widely used in building materials, it has made its way into literally every building, factory, home, and farm in the United States.

Chapter 2

Asbestos Disease

How does asbestos cause disease? The answer to this question is not fully understood by medical scientists. This much is known: During various industrial operations, countless numbers of invisible asbestos fibers can become airborne in the manner of house dust. Because of their tiny size, these needle-like fibers are easily inhaled and swallowed. Although many asbestos particles are eliminated from the body through natural processes, many others find their way into the lungs and respiratory tracts of exposed workers. Here they can become lodged in delicate tissues, causing lesions that eventually result in disease.

Because of its remarkable durability, asbestos can remain in the lungs and other tissues for a lifetime. Moreover, since asbestos fibers can be transported by the blood stream and the lymphatic system, they can migrate from the lungs, causing disease in other parts of the body.

People do not become sick immediately after inhaling asbestos. The delay from the time of first exposure to the time asbestos disease develops in known as the latent period. For most asbestos disease, this latent period is anywhere from 15 to 35 or more years.

What kinds of disease are caused by asbestos?

Heavy exposure to asbestos can cause asbestosis, and greatly increases the risk of lung cancer, and cancer of the gastrointestinal tract. Even lighter exposure to the mineral can result in mesothelioma, a cancer of the membranes that encase the lungs and line the abdominal cavity.

- **Asbestosis.** This chronic disease is characterized by fibrosis (scarring) of the lungs as a result of inhalation and retention of asbestos fibers. Asbestosis usually occurs in workers who have been heavily exposed to asbestos dust. The earliest and most prominent sign of asbestosis is shortness of breath during exertion. However, this symptom rarely becomes apparent until at least 10 years after first exposure to the mineral. By then the disease is often in an advanced state.

A characteristic sign of asbestosis is a dry-crackling sound (rales) which may be heard on examination of the lungs during inhalation. Clubbing, or thickening, of the fingers occasionally occurs in the late stages of the disease. X-ray examination reveals scarring of the lungs as asbestosis develops. Lung functions tests show impairment of the maximum volume of air an afflicted worker can inhale.

Asbestosis is an insidious and progressive disease. This is because asbestos, being a mineral, is virtually indestructible in lung tissue. Once inhaled, it continues to react within the lungs for a lifetime. Many people with asbestosis develop cor pulmonale—right-sided heart failure—which is often the cause of death among such patients.

During the first 40 years of this century, more asbestos workers died of asbestosis than of any other asbestos-induced disease. As factory dust levels were lowered, however, the attack rate of severe asbestosis was slowed. As a result, instead of dying of asbestosis, asbestos workers began living long enough to develop asbestos-induced cancer.

- **Lung cancer and gastrointestinal cancer.** Lung cancer is by far the most common cause of death among asbestos workers today, particularly among those who smoke cigarettes. Between 20 and 25 percent of all deaths in some groups of heavily exposed workers are due to lung cancer. By comparison, about 4 to 5 percent of all deaths in the general population are caused by lung cancer.

Asbestos inhalation combined with cigarette smoking

greatly increases the risk of developing lung cancer. Investigators at the Mount Sinai School of Medicine in New York City have found that asbestos workers who smoke run an 8-times greater risk of developing lung cancer than smokers in the general population who do not work with asbestos.

Asbestos workers who smoke cigarettes are between *60* and *90* times more likely to die of lung cancer than men who neither work with asbestos nor smoke.

About 10 percent of all asbestos workers die of cancer of the gastrointestinal tract, which includes cancer of the stomach, esophagus, colon, and rectum. Of these, only the risk of developing esophageal cancer is increased by cigarette smoking.

No one knows how much asbestos exposure is necessary to cause lung cancer and gastrointestinal cancer. However, a study of 250 asbestos workers who were heavily exposed to asbestos dust for periods of only three months or less shows that 25 years later they died of lung cancer at 3.5 times the expected rate. Some investigators consider it possible that a worker who was heavily exposed to asbestos for just one day could develop cancer years later as a result.

- **Mesothelioma.** This type of cancer attacks the pleura, which is the delicate membrane that encases the lungs. It also attacks the peritoneum, a similar membrane that lines the abdominal cavity. Twenty-five years ago, mesothelioma was so rare it was considered to be a pathological curiosity. Today, more than 5 percent of all asbestos workers die of this disease.

Mesothelioma takes from 20 to 50 years to develop. Cigarette smoking does not appear to be a factor. Remarkably, mesothelioma almost never occurs without some, even if slight, history of exposure to asbestos. For this reason, medical researchers have come to consider mesothelioma a "marker" disease for asbestos exposure.

Mesothelioma is more than an occupational disease. It is now being found increasingly in people whose only known exposure to asbestos was that they lived in the vicinity of factories where asbestos products were manufactured, or lived in the same house as workers who came home with asbestos dust on their clothes.

Mesothelioma is almost always malignant, and, when malignant, is invariably fatal.

Chapter 3

A History of Asbestos Disease

The first victim of asbestos disease may well have been a Stone Age potter who pulverized asbestos-containing rock to obtain fibers for reinforcing his clay. Or it may have been one of his ancestors whose exposure occurred from living in a cave hollowed out of asbestos-bearing rock. However, the first mention of asbestos disease does not occur until around the time of Christ, when a sickness of the lungs was reportedly observed in slaves whose occupation was to weave asbestos into cloth.

Nearly 2000 years were to pass before the health hazard posed by asbestos came to light again!

Modern knowledge of asbestos disease dates from the year 1899, when an autopsy performed on the body of a 33-year-old asbestos worker in London revealed severe scarring of the lungs. This man was the last survivor of a group of 10 men (all of whom died in their thirties) who had worked in the carding room of an asbestos textile factory.

A few years later, it was reported that 50 French workers had died of lung disease after only 5 years of exposure to asbestos in an asbestos weaving mill in Calvados.

On this side of the Atlantic, asbestos was also becoming an occupational hazard. Indeed, by World War I the records of some American insurance companies showed increased mortality among asbestos workers. As a result, these companies were often reluctant to insure asbestos workers.

The first official case of death due to asbestos disease appeared in the medical literature in 1924. It was reported by Dr. W. E. Cooke, an English physician, who later called the disease asbestosis. Cooke's discovery provided the point of departure for hundreds of investigations of asbestos disease that have been conducted during the past 55 years.

In 1929, a study of English asbestos textile workers performed by Dr. E. R. A. Merewether, a medical inspector of the British Government, showed that more than one in four were suffering from asbestosis. As a result, Parliament passed legislation in 1931 that made asbestosis a compensable disease, and that required improved ventilation and dust control in asbestos textile factories.

Unfortunately, no such preventive measures were taken in the United States. However, the suggestion that asbestos could cause malignant disease was first raised in 1935 by two American doctors, Kenneth M. Lynch and W. A. Smith, who noticed an association between asbestosis and lung cancer. The link between asbestos exposure and lung cancer was definitely established in 1955 by Dr. Richard S. Doll, of the British Medical Research Council. He demonstrated that the risk of lung cancer in a group of asbestos textile workers with more than 20 years of exposure was 11 times as great as that of men in the general population.

By 1960, asbestos was recognized as the cause of mesothelioma. This came about when a South African pathologist named J. Christopher Wagner discovered several dozen cases of this rare and fatal tumor among people whose only exposure to asbestos consisted of living in the vicinity of asbestos mills and dumps. Dr. Wagner's finding was the first suggestion that the asbestos health hazard might be environmental as well as occupational. Additional evidence soon came from England and the United States, where mesothelioma was found among people who had simply lived in the home of an asbestos worker, or who had lived near an asbestos factory.

During 1962, Dr. Irving J. Selikoff, of New York City's Mount Sinai Medical School, and Dr. E. Cuyler Hammond, of the American Cancer Society, conducted a pioneer study of the mortality experience of a group of insulation workers who had been exposed to asbestos for more than 20 years. The results were alarming to say the least. Excess death among these men was 25 percent greater than what could have been expected to occur in the general population. The reason was not hard to come by. Nearly 50 percent of the insulation workers were dying of asbestos-related disease, including asbestosis, lung cancer, gastrointestinal cancer, and mesothelioma.

This study furnished the first absolute proof that industrial exposure to asbestos was extremely hazardous. It was published in the spring of 1964 in the *Journal of the American Medical Association,* and was delivered at the Conference on the Biological Effects of Asbestos in October of that year.

A milestone conference

The 1964 meeting was the first conference to deal with the broad spectrum of problems associated with human exposure to asbestos. For this reason, it proved to be a milestone in the long scientific journey that had begun 40 years before, when Dr. Cooke described the first clear case of asbestosis.

In addition to evidence of the terrible cancer death rate among American asbestos insulation workers, the 1964 conference brought to light many other facts. The sad plight of the American asbestos workers was also found in the asbestos workers of Dresden, in East Germany. Mesotheliomas were reported among British shipyard workers who had received only light or intermittent exposure to asbestos dust. Dr. Wagner reported on the mesotheliomas he had found in South Africa in people who had not actually worked with asbestos, but merely lived in the vicinity of asbestos mines and mills. And Dr. Muriel L. Newhouse reported on cases of mesothelioma she had found among the relatives of asbestos workers in London.

At the 1964 meeting, the American asbestos industry was severely criticized for trying to deny that asbestos exposure could cause lung cancer and mesothelioma. An industry spokesman claimed that there was too much pessimism about asbestos at the conference.

Dr. J. C. Gilson, of the Medical Research Council, Llandough Hospital, in Wales, gave a final overview of the proceedings. He said, "It is abundantly clear from the evidence presented at the Conference that in future much greater care must be taken to eliminate unnecessary exposure to asbestos dust wherever it occurs."

The sad price of neglect

The 1964 conference amounted to a grand jury indictment of asbestos as a major threat to human health. At that time, however, the public and the Congress were only just beginning to realize the necessity for controlling occupational and environmental health hazards such as asbestos. And, without the necessary public and congressional pressure, government health agencies were not motivated to deal adequately with the problem. As a result, the asbestos hazard was neglected for nearly a decade longer. Here is what happened:

- Vast amounts of asbestos fireproofing material continued to be sprayed on the steel girders of high-rise buildings. This practice contaminated the air of virtually every American city with asbestos fibers, and posed an unknown health hazard for millions of unsuspecting urban dwellers. At the same time, hundreds of thousands of construction workers were indirectly exposed to dangerous amounts of asbestos dust by virtue of working in the vicinity of asbestos-spraying operations.
- Asbestos materials continued to be widely used in soundproof ceilings and walls in school buildings throughout the nation. Because of wear and tear, asbestos fibers soon began to contaminate the air that many school children were breathing.
- Little or nothing was done to control asbestos dust in shipyards, especially during refitting procedures when asbestos insulation was ripped out and replaced. As a result, thousands of shipyard workers continued to be exposed to hazardous amounts of asbestos dust.
- Many in the asbestos industry continued to deny that asbestos could cause lung cancer and mesothelioma. Industry made inadequate efforts to control asbestos-dust exposures in

> its plants and factories. As a result, asbestos workers in the United States could sometimes be found working in clouds of dust that obscured the light.

During the 1960s, state and Federal health agencies failed to protect the health of American asbestos workers by neglecting to enforce even the inadequate asbestos dust control measures that were then in effect. And they made little or no effort to educate workers about the health risks of asbestos exposure.

Even after Congress passed the Occupational Safety and Health Act of 1970, these agencies were slow to enforce the new and tougher regulations that were issued for asbestos exposure.

Because of such neglect, many injured asbestos workers and the relatives of those who had died of asbestos disease began to seek remedy through litigation. During the early 1970s, the number of asbestos lawsuits in the United States increased dramatically. Today, the American asbestos industry faces liabilities estimated to be in the billions of dollars. Moreover, because of its own failure to protect the health of asbestos workers, the Federal government has already been a defendant in an asbestos lawsuit. In fact, the government has agreed to pay nearly $6 million to former workers in an asbestos insulation factory that had operated in Tyler, Texas.

But this is the price of neglect in mere dollars. The real price is the awful death toll and human suffering experienced by the nation's asbestos workers and their families. No one really knows how great this toll will prove to be. However, some researchers believe that between two and four million American men and women may die of asbestos-related disease.

Part II
THE ORDEAL OF THE WORLD'S ASBESTOS WORKERS

Asbestos is a common mineral found in many countries of the world. It has several thousand industrial uses. It is mined, milled, and fabricated into various products by hundreds of thousands of workers, and it is utilized in one way or another by millions of others.

Many, if not most, of these workers run some risk of developing asbestos disease. No one knows just how much of a risk for there are many factors that must be taken into consideration. One thing, however, is certain: Wherever it has been found, and wherever it has been used, asbestos has proved to be a serious occupational health hazard.

The following chapters give some idea of the immense amount of medical detective work that has gone into following the trail of asbestos disease among various groups of workers throughout the world.

Chapter 4

The Insulation Workers

Asbestos was used as an insulation material as early as 1866. The first insulation workers' union was formed in New York City in 1883. Known as the "Salamander Association of Boiler and Pipe Felters," the group derived its odd name from a practical joke that was played on Marco Polo. It seems that in the latter half of the 13th century, when the Venetian traveller was crossing a part of Siberia then known as the Great Empire of Tartary, he was shown some cloth that would not burn, and was told by his Tartar hosts that it was made from salamander's wool.

In 1910, the Salamander Association merged with other independent insulation locals and was chartered by the American Federation of Labor (AFL) as the International Association of Heat and Frost Insulators and Asbestos Workers. Today, the members of this union are primarily employed in the building trades on construction work. Some of them also work as insulators in refineries, industrial facilities, shipyards, and power plants.

Until the early 1940s, the molded pipe coverings, asbestos cement, and asbestos felt and paper products used by the insulation workers contained only chrysotile asbestos. Virtually all of this chrysotile was imported into the United States from Canada. During the 1930s, small quantities of amosite asbestos began to be imported from South Africa. Amosite was widely used as insulation in American shipyards during World War II.

By and large, the asbestos exposure of the insulation workers is believed to have been comparatively light and intermittent. One reason for this is that the asbestos content of most of the insulation materials they used was less than 20 percent. Another reason was that much of the work they performed was done out-of-doors. Occasionally, however, these men worked in tight quarters, especially in shipyards where they ripped out and replaced old asbestos insulation in the confines of boiler rooms and submarine hulls. Also, it seems likely that many asbestos-insulation workers have been exposed from time to time to very high levels of asbestos dust for short periods. Some researchers are concerned that such peak exposures could play an important role in the development of asbestos disease.

Until the mid-1960s, few dust counts were made in areas where asbestos insulation work was being performed. Retrospective analysis and extrapolation suggests, however, that the insulation workers may have been exposed to dust levels that averaged between 4 and 12 fibers in each cubic centimeter of air. This is approximately the volume contained in a thimbleful. It is a dust level that was considered for many years to be perfectly safe for human exposure.

Such is no longer the case.

Death among the insulation workers

Thanks to Dr. Irving J. Selikoff and his colleagues at New York City's Mount Sinai School of Medicine, and to Dr. E. Cuyler Hammond, of the American Cancer Society, the mortality experience of the asbestos insulation workers has been documented with great care and precision.

In their 1962 study, Drs. Selikoff and Hammond traced a group of 632 asbestos insulation workers in the New York–New Jersey metropolitan area. These men had been on the union rolls in 1943, and had been exposed to chrysotile asbestos dust for 20 years or more. During the first 10 years of observation (1943–52), there was no particular excess in total deaths among this group. But once 20 years had passed since these men were first exposed to asbestos, a grim picture emerged.

According to the standard mortality rates in the United States, 195 deaths were expected to occur among them. Instead, there were 253. The excess deaths were due to asbestosis and asbestos-related cancer.

- 42 of the insulation workers died of lung cancer—7 times the expected rate.
- Gastrointestinal cancer claimed 29 lives—approximately 3 times as many as expected.
- Mesothelioma, an almost unknown disease in the general population, killed 7 men.
- In addition, there were 12 deaths from asbestosis.

The disaster continues

Since 1962, Drs. Selikoff and Hammond have continued to study this group of asbestos workers. By the end of 1976, a broad picture of the asbestos-disease toll among them had become tragically clear. Nineteen percent of these men were dying of lung cancer. Nine percent were dying of gastrointestinal cancer. Eight percent were succumbing to mesothelioma. And 9 percent were being killed by asbestosis and other noninfectious lung disease.

Thus, fully 45 percent of the original group of 632 asbestos insulation workers exposed to chrysotile asbestos in the New York–New Jersey metropolitan area are known to have died of asbestos-related disease.

The same grim mortality pattern has held true for men who joined the union after 1943. It is interesting to note that these men were exposed to both chrysotile and amosite asbestos. The fact that they experienced essentially the same disease and death rate as their predecessors indicates that amosite may not be even more carcinogenic than chrysotile, as some researchers had predicted.

The disaster spreads

It should come as no surprise that the tragic death and disease toll among the metropolitan insulation workers has been found among asbestos insulation workers elsewhere. Dr. Selikoff, Dr. Hammond and their colleagues have been studying 17,800 men who were members of the asbestos workers union in the United States and Canada at the beginning of 1967.

Their methods of observation have been exact and painstaking. Whenever one of these workers dies, the Mount Sinai group is notified, and a death certificate is forwarded. Additional information is then obtained for each death, including clinical data, X-ray pictures, pathological specimens and autopsy findings.

During the 10-year period from the beginning of 1967 to the end of 1976, only a limited amount of excess disease occurred among workers who had been exposed to asbestos dust for less than 20 years. But among the 12,051 insulation workers who reached the 20-year period since first exposure to asbestos, the catastrophic pattern was repeated.

According to the standard mortality tables, 1,376 deaths were expected to occur among these men. Instead, there were 1,946. There were 160 deaths from asbestosis; 912 men died of cancer, and 450 of these were from lung cancer. This was more than 4.5 times the expected rate. Gastrointestinal cancer continued to occur at about 3 times the normal rate. And there were 170 deaths from mesothelioma.

Some grim conclusions

As it happens, the vast majority of these 17,800 American and Canadian insulation workers were exposed to asbestos long before the terrible cancer-producing potential of the mineral was fully and properly appreciated. It also happens that the present standards for exposure to asbestos dust in the United States and Canada are largely based upon criteria designed to prevent asbestosis.

Yet, as can clearly be seen from the awful mortality experience of the insulation workers, the major killer of these men is not asbestosis, but cancer. In fact, cancer is killing between 35 percent and 40 percent of the insulation workers!

Since most occupational cancer experts acknowledge that there is *no* known safe level of exposure to a cancer-causing substance, two conclusions can be drawn as a result of the mortality studies of the insulation workers.

The first is that the insulation workers are still being exposed to hazardous amounts of asbestos. The second is that the price of this exposure will be paid in excess disease and death among these men 20 to 40 years from now.

Chapter 5

Miners and Millers

Canada and the Soviet Union produce 90 percent of the world's asbestos although the mineral is mined in dozens of other countries. Chrysotile, the most common variety, accounts for 95 percent of all commercially produced asbestos. It is mined in Canada, the Soviet Union, the United States, South Africa, Rhodesia, Australia, Brazil, China, Columbia, Cyprus, Italy, Japan, Mexico, Switzerland, and Yugoslavia. South Africa is the leading producer of amosite and crocidolite asbestos. All asbestos except chrysotile is taken from underground mines. Most chrysotile is produced by open pit mining. Asbestos disease has been reported among miners and millers in Canada, South Africa, Finland, Cyprus, Australia, and the Soviet Union.

Mining and milling in Canada

Chrysotile asbestos was first mined in 1878 in the Eastern Townships region of Quebec, some 100 miles east of Montreal. Since then dozens of companies have produced asbestos fiber from this area. The two principal mining centers are the towns of Asbestos and Thetford. By 1966, a total of some 28,000 people had worked in the Quebec asbestos mines and mills.

Most asbestos mining operations in Quebec are of the open pit type. In this process, 40-foot holes are drilled in asbestos-containing ore deposits. The holes are then charged with explosives and blasted. Afterward, the loose ore is loaded onto trucks and transported to a crushing machine. The crusher breaks rocks up to four feet in diameter into pieces 6 inches or less in size. Additional crushing further reduces the dimensions of these fragments. Moisture is then removed by heating the crushed ore in huge dryers.

During milling operations, the ore goes through various stages of screening and vacuum separation in which loose asbestos fiber is air-lifted from the host rock. Ore and fiber are transported throughout the mills by conveyor belts, chutes, and vacuum-exhausted pipes.

Most of the workforce in the Quebec asbestos industry is employed in the mills. Laborers perform general clean-up by sweeping or shovelling up asbestos fiber that has spilled from the processing equipment. They also feed asbestos into fiber storage bins. Floor walkers continually monitor the operation of machinery and the movement of fiber throughout the mills. One of their tasks is to clear up stoppages of fiber flow. Maintenance personnel include machinists, millwrights, sheetmetal workers, and electricians.

Before 1970, asbestos fiber concentrations were not measured separately in the Quebec mines and mills. Instead, total dust counts were made, which included nonasbestos dust from the ore that was being crushed, dried, and processed. Crude estimates based upon limited data indicate that virtually all jobs in this industry were very dusty in times past. Some jobs were far dustier than others. For example, workers used to prepare asbestos fiber for shipment by shovelling it into burlap bags. This task is now accomplished by automatic bagging machines.

In spite of greatly improved dust-control measures, air samples taken in 1973-75 show that many of the workers in the Quebec asbestos mines and mills are still being exposed to significant concentrations of asbestos fiber at various times during their work. Exposures of people working in the drying and crushing operations are generally highest. Fiber counts in the milling process tend to be somewhat lower. However, average dust concentrations in most work categories greatly exceeded the asbestos standard of 5 fibers per cubic centimeter of air then in effect in the United States.

Death among Canadian miners and millers

A few years ago, Dr. William J. Nicholson, Dr. Selikoff, and their colleagues at the Mount Sinai School of Medicine undertook a study of mortality in Canadian miners and millers exposed to chrysotile asbestos. One purpose of the investigation was to determine whether exposure to chrysotile asbestos alone could cause serious disease. Another was to compare the death rate among the Canadian miners and millers with that of other workers who were exposed to chrysotile fibers, either in factories making asbestos products or by using or installing the products themselves.

The Mount Sinai investigators studied a group of 544 employees who had spent at least 20 years working in the mines and mills in the Thetford area. Work histories were obtained through interviews with each man who was alive in 1973.

Sixteen percent of the deaths among these 544 men were from lung cancer. Fifteen percent were caused by asbestosis. Excess deaths from these two diseases accounted for 43 out of 178 deaths in the study group.

Overall, the 544 Canadian miners and millers experienced less excess mortality than either asbestos insulators or factory workers. A chief reason for this was that there was only one death from mesothelioma among these men.

Some researchers believe that this finding indicates that despite its effect in causing lung cancer and asbestosis, chrysotile exposure has less influence on the development of mesothelioma. However, Dr. Nicholson has suggested that the lesser mesothelioma risk experienced by the miners and millers may be explained by the fact that the greatest percentage of longer and thicker asbestos fibers would occur in their work environment, whereas shorter and thinner fibers would be expected to occur in the work environment of asbestos insulators and factory workers. These smaller fibers can, of course, be more easily inhaled. They can also be transported readily to the periphery of the lung and become lodged in the pleural membrane that encases it.

Another study of chrysotile exposure in Canada

In 1966, Dr. J. Corbett McDonald and colleagues from

McGill University in Montreal undertook to study mortality in Canadian miners and millers. They did so at the invitation of the Canadian government, which was concerned about reports of disease among asbestos workers in other parts of the world.

The McGill researchers selected a group of 11,788 workers who had been born between 1891 and 1920, and who had worked in mines and mills near the towns of Asbestos and Thetford. These employees were characterized on the basis of a dust-exposure index (low, medium, high, and very high), and according to duration of employment. The average asbestos-dust exposure was estimated from previous dust measurements and approximations.

Dr. McDonald and his colleagues found that the mortality experience in the whole study group compared favorably with that of the general population of Quebec Province. However, deaths from asbestosis occurred 5 times more frequently in the most heavily exposed group of men than in all the other categories. A 20 percent excess of deaths was observed in this group. Moreover, the men with very heavy exposure developed lung cancer at 5 times the rate of men with low exposure.

The McGill investigators concluded that "The major occupational hazard of chrysotile asbestos exposure are respiratory cancer and the complications of pulmonary asbestosis."

Another theory concerning mesothelioma

Dr. McDonald and his assistants observed only 12 deaths from mesothelioma out of a total of 4,547 deaths in their study group of miners and millers. Previously they had conducted a study in which they observed 9 deaths from mesothelioma in a group of only 199 factory workers who had been exposed to crocidolite asbestos in the manufacture of military gas masks. Because of this they have concluded that exposure to crocidolite carries a far greater risk of mesothelioma than does exposure to chrysotile.

Some comparisons and conclusions

The excess death rate from asbestos disease among the Canadian miners and millers studied by the McGill researchers is apparently far less than the rate found in a smaller group of men from the same industry by the Mount Sinai investigators. However, it is interesting to note that the death rate among the 544 employees in the Mount Sinai study group is very similar to the death rate experienced by the most heavily exposed group in the McGill study.

A relationship between heavy asbestos dust exposure and serious disease and death certainly appears to exist among the chrysotile miners and millers. However, dust indexes that do not indicate the actual prevalence of asbestos fibers, as well as fiber exposure levels based upon estimates of past conditions, do not provide a sound basis for establishing occupational exposure standards for the prevention of asbestos disease in the future.

Much work remains to be done on the complicated dose-response relationships governing the development of asbestosis, lung cancer, and mesothelioma. Studies should be undertaken to resolve the question of whether some types of asbestos fiber can cause mesothelioma more readily than others. The role of fiber size in the development of this disease should also be thoroughly investigated.

Conditions in South Africa

Crocidolite asbestos was first mined in South Africa in 1893. Amosite mining began in 1916. Today, South Africa is the world's leading producer of amosite and crocidolite. The country has about 30 asbestos mines in operation, each with one or more asbestos mills. Twenty thousand workers are exposed to asbestos but there is a high turnover so that the total population at risk over time is much higher.

During 1949, the Department of Mines of South Africa carried out an X-ray and clinical survey of people working in the asbestos fields. Asbestosis was found in a large number of these workers, many of whom had been employed in the mines and mills for a long time. Little effort was made in those days to control asbestos dust-exposure levels, which are reported to have been extraordinarily high. As a result, asbestosis was found to be developing in South African miners and millers with only 5 or 6 years of exposure.

The doctor who made the first official survey of health conditions in the asbestos fields of South Africa reported that industrial hygiene in the mines and mills was deplorable. He later described young Bantu children as spending their days inside large jute shipping bags, where they were forced by overseers armed with whips to trample down fluffy amosite asbestos as it came cascading down over their heads into the bags. He found that some of these children had developed asbestosis with cor pulmonale (right-sided heart failure) before the age of 12. For this reason, he stated that he would be very surprised if any of them had lived long enough to develop either lung cancer or mesothelioma.

Although all mines in South Africa were placed under statutory control in 1953, dust levels were not significantly reduced until 1964. Not surprisingly, therefore, lung disease is prevalent among South African workers today. A recent study shows that lung abnormalities such as thickening of the pleural membrane have been detected in nearly 50 percent of the workers who have had more than 15 years of exposure. Similar abnormalities have been found in people living near asbestos mines and mills in Finland.

The authors of the South African study report that pleural thickening does not appear to depend upon asbestos fiber concentrations, but on duration of exposure and on time that has elapsed since first exposure. They theorize that pleural abnormality may be caused by submicroscopic fibers too small to be measured. If it proves to be true, this suggestion could be tremendously important because most asbestos exposure standards, including the one now in effect in the United States, completely ignore the disease potential of smaller fibers.

All working miners in South Africa are given annual physical examinations. Compensation is provided at the first detectable stage of asbestosis. Nonetheless, there is little or no medical follow-up of people who have left the industry. Consequently, knowledge about the overall mortality experience of South African asbestos workers is scanty, and the authorities have no idea of the rate of lung cancer and mesothelioma among them.

In general, the South African authorities appear to have more fully investigated the incidence of asbestosis in their miners and millers than the incidence of lung cancer and other malignant disease. However, the significant number of mesotheliomas found in the 1950s among people who simply lived in the vicinity of South African asbestos mines and mills indicates that this disease can be expected to occur in people with industrial exposure as well.

Little information is available at this time on the health experience of black workers in South Africa, who are believed to have been exposed to the highest concentrations of asbestos dust. Studies of disease among black workers are now said to be under way. Such studies may provide a clearer picture of the total incidence of asbestos-related cancer among the miners and millers in South Africa.

Chapter 6
The Factory Workers

Asbestos disease began to take its toll of asbestos textile factory workers at the turn of the century. This was about 20 years after asbestos began to be used in industry. Industrial hygiene was virtually unknown in those days, however, and nothing was done to control dust levels. In 1931, after it was learned that one in four asbestos textile workers was suffering from asbestosis, the British Parliament passed legislation requiring improved ventilation and dust control in British asbestos factories.

Here in the United States, no such action was taken. Yet as early as World War I, some American insurance companies were reluctant to insure asbestos workers because of their excess death rate. American asbestos workers continued to work in unsafe conditions for many more decades. Indeed, as recently as 1971, some asbestos factory employees in the United States, such as those who worked in the infamous Tyler, Texas, insulation plant, were toiling in clouds of asbestos dust that obscured the light!

This chapter describes the sad plight of asbestos factory workers on both sides of the Atlantic and elsewhere in the world.

London, England

Dr. Muriel L. Newhouse, of the London School of Hygiene and Tropical Medicine, has investigated the health situation at an East London factory where asbestos textiles and insulation materials were manufactured. The plant operated from 1913 until 1968, and the workers were exposed to all three major varieties of asbestos—chrysotile, crocidolite, and amosite.

Among a group of male workers in this factory, many more deaths occurred than had been expected on the basis of the standard mortality rates for Great Britain. About 20 percent of the men died from lung cancer, and 10 percent from mesothelioma. Cancer of the lung and pleura occurred at 5 times the expected rate in those with heavy exposure.

More than 400 of the 922 women who worked at the factory between 1936 and 1942 were employed in the asbestos textile departments. One hundred women worked as mattress makers. Crocidolite was used in the textile department and exposure to dust was estimated to have been very heavy.

There was a great excess of cancer of the lung and pleura in the women who were heavily exposed over a long period of time. These women also experienced excess cancer of the breast and ovary. As with the men, approximately 10 percent of them died of mesothelioma.

It was obvious that men and women who began working in this factory in their early twenties had a markedly diminished life expectancy.

Paterson, New Jersey

Just before the United States entered World War II, an amosite asbestos factory was established in Paterson to supply the Navy with asbestos insulation for the pipes, boilers, and turbines of its ships. From June 1941 through December 1945, 933 men worked in this plant, which continued to operate until 1954.

Because of wartime conditions, many of these men left employment to enter the Armed Services, or drifted off to other work after a short stay on the job. No dust counts were taken in the factory, but the ventilation system is known to have been extremely poor, and it is presumed that the asbestos fiber concentrations were very high.

Thus many of the 933 workers in the Paterson factory sustained intense exposure to amosite asbestos over a relatively short period of time.

When investigators from the Mount Sinai School of Medicine studied the mortality experience of these 933 men, they uncovered a disaster similar to the one that befell the asbestos insulation workers. By 1974, 200 excess deaths had occurred among the Paterson factory workers. This is why:

- The death rate from lung cancer was 7 times the expected rate.
- Twice as many men died of gastrointestinal cancer as was expected.
- 10 men died of mesothelioma.
- 25 men died of asbestosis.
- All in all, 117 deaths occurred from asbestos-related cancer.

More recently, the Mount Sinai investigators have studied the Paterson factory workers according to duration of exposure to amosite asbestos. Some of these men worked for as little as one day. Others were employed for one or more months. Still others worked for a year or more. And a few men worked at the plant during the entire 13 years it was in operation.

It used to be believed that only heavy exposure to asbestos over a long period of time could cause significant disease. Because of the Paterson worker study, however, such opinions must now be revised.

Thirty-five years after first exposure, the men who worked in the Paterson factory for only one month or less are dying of lung cancer *three* times more frequently than other men in New Jersey! And the men who worked two years or more are dying of the same disease at 6 times the expected rate.

The sad experience of the Paterson factory workers clearly shows that even short-term asbestos exposure can be extremely hazardous. The reason for this is that inhaled asbestos fibers can work within the delicate tissues of the lungs to cause malignant disease over a very long period of time.

Manville, New Jersey

Workers at another asbestos factory in New Jersey have also experienced a health disaster. One of the largest asbestos plants in the world is located in Manville. The mortality experience of the 1,348 men who retired from this factory between 1941 and 1967 was studied from 1941 to 1973. During this time, these men had an overall death rate that was 20 percent higher than that of other men in the general population of the United States.

Not surprisingly, this excess was found to be caused almost entirely by cancer and diseases of the respiratory system.

Naharihya, Israel

Asbestos has no respect for frontiers or nationalities. In 1953, an asbestos cement products plant began operating in Naharihya. Water and sewage pipe, as well as sheets for walls and ceilings, were the chief products. Crocidolite and chrysotile asbestos were used in their manufacture.

Since 1953, a total of 3,608 workers were employed at this factory. As early as 1967, they were found to be dying of cancer more than twice as often as other Israelis. For this reason, dust-control measures were established in the factory. Nevertheless, Israeli health authorities expect that when more time has passed the cancer rate among these workers will rise.

Some sobering conclusions

Asbestos factory workers in the United States, England, and elsewhere in the world have long been exposed to excessive levels of asbestos dust. This has resulted in a death rate among them that can only be described as disastrous.

What can be done to prevent this awful death toll? Reducing exposure can, of course, delay the occurrence of asbestos disease. It can also reduce the frequency with which disease occurs. Unfortunately, recent studies of asbestos factory workers show that the disease potential of asbestos fibers continues long after direct exposure to asbestos has ceased. In fact, it continues for as long as asbestos fibers remain in lung tissue, which means for a lifetime. Thus excess deaths in asbestos workers tend to become more pronounced as the years go by.

It is sobering to consider that disease in asbestos workers

today is the result of exposures that in many cases took place 30 or 40 years ago. Since then, the use of asbestos has increased tremendously. And with it, of course, the risk of wider exposure to workers and people in the general population.

Many medical scientists believe that exposure standards for asbestos workers are still too high. They point out that there is no known safe level of exposure for a known carcinogen. They also point out that workers in enclosed factory areas are particularly at risk of inhaling significant quantities of asbestos dust.

What will the death toll among asbestos factory workers be in the 21st century? The answer to this question rests in the preventive measures we take today.

Chapter 7
The Shipyard Problem

Asbestos has been used to insulate the steam pipes and boilers of ships since the turn of the century. Sometimes the fiber is woven into a mattress or cloth and wrapped around high-pressure piping. In other instances, it is applied as a cementitious and easily crumbled material called boiler composition. This consists of a powder of 85 percent magnesia and 15 percent asbestos, which is mixed with water to form a thick paste. In some shipyards, asbestos has been sprayed as fireproofing on bulkheads and on the undersides of decks.

Shipyard worker populations tend to fluctuate greatly. For example, in 1918 there were 318,500 shipyard workers in the United States. This number decreased after World War I, and the workforce averaged about 75,000 during the 1920s and 1930s.

With the approach of World War II, American shipyards underwent a tremendous expansion as this nation undertook to build and repair ships for the free world. Total employment in United States shipyards rose from 168,000 in June 1940 to 1,722,500 by December 1943. In some yards between 10 and 20 percent of these workers were women. The turnover was very high, averaging more than 100 percent annually. It is estimated that about 4.5 million men and women were employed in United States naval and civilian shipyards during World War II.

After 1945, the number of shipyard workers rapidly decreased. For the past 25 years or so, the workforce has remained stable at about 200,000 workers.

Asbestos exposure in shipyards

The most important aspect of asbestos exposure in shipyards is the character of the workforce at risk. In 1943, one in 500 workers in private shipyards in the United States was an actual "asbestos worker." The other 499 worked as welders, shipfitters, machinists, pipefitters, electricians, carpenters, laborers, painters, sheetmetal workers, riggers, and so forth. Few precautions were taken in those days to avoid asbestos exposure. Therefore, during shipboard asbestos operations, many of these workers sustained heavy exposure to asbestos dust for short periods of time in small, poorly ventilated compartments. What they experienced is called indirect occupational exposure.

Since no dust counts were taken, no one really knows what levels of asbestos fiber existed in shipyards during World War II. However, there is good reason to believe that they were sometimes very high. Ten years ago, an investigation of the Royal Navy ship repair yards at Devonport, England, showed alarming levels of asbestos dust during the application of asbestos materials on pipes and boilers. In fact, in some work areas the asbestos fiber concentration was too dense to count. The highest count in this survey was more than 3,000 fibers per cubic centimeter of air.

That was *1500* times higher than the occupational standard for asbestos exposure in England today!

Asbestos disease in British shipyard workers

With such high levels of exposure, it is small wonder that asbestos disease began to afflict British shipyard workers. The British shipbuilding and ship repair industry was reactivated in 1935, 5 or 6 years before a similar expansion took place in the United States. Cases of mesothelioma were first reported among shipyard workers in Belfast and Liverpool in the late 1950s and early 1960s. This is consistent, of course, with the latent period for the development of this tumor, which is between 20 and 40 years.

In 1968, Dr. Peter Harries, a Surgeon Commander in the Royal Navy, reported five cases of pleural mesothelioma among civilian employees of the dockyard at Devonport. None of these patients was an asbestos worker. One was a boilermaker; another was a shipwright; and a third was a laborer. The two other victims were a pipefitter and a welder. These workers could only have been exposed to asbestos as unsuspecting bystanders. The fact that they had developed mesothelioma meant that thousands upon thousands of shipyard workers the world over might be at risk of contracting this disease.

Cases of mesothelioma in the Devonport-Plymouth area now total 103. One hundred of them have been associated either with work in the dockyard or with service in naval vessels. In addition, a considerable amount of pulmonary fibrosis is developing in men whose exposure was intermittent and spread over many years. It is estimated that 50 percent of the total workforce of 15,000 men in the Devenport shipyard have been exposed intermittently to asbestos by virtue of having worked in the vicinity of various asbestos operations.

Some alarming corroboration

Even more disturbing are recent data from shipyards in Barrow-in-Furness that have been collected and published by Dr. John Edge of High Carley Hospital. Between 1964 and 1971, 429 of the Barrow shipyard workers showed X-ray evidence of having developed a condition called pleural plaque. This is a thickening of the pleural membrane often associated with exposure to asbestos.

Dr. Edge undertook to compare the mortality experience of these workers with a control group of 429 men of matched ages from the neighboring city of Carlisle, who showed no signs of pleural plaque upon X-ray examination. The results were depressing.

By the end of 1976, there were 127 deaths among the 429 men with pleural plaque, as compared to only 74 deaths among the 429 men in the control group without this condition. The excess was primarily due to 19 deaths from lung cancer and 23 deaths from mesothelioma which occurred among the shipyard workers. Among the control group of men from Carlisle, only 4 men died of lung cancer, while none died of mesothelioma.

Mesothelioma in the Netherlands

During 1968, 25 cases of mesothelioma were reported on the island of Walcheren in the Netherlands; 22 of these cases occurred among people who were employed at the Royal "de Schelde" shipyard in Vlissingen. Once again, these mesothelioma victims were workers with only indirect occupational exposure to asbestos.

When these disturbing findings were reported by Dr. J. Stumphius, chief medical officer of the shipyard, the Dutch authorities acted with commendable speed. Royal "de Schelde" stopped the use of all asbestos insulation in 1970. Ships now under construction there for the Royal Dutch Navy are practically asbestos-free.

Royal "de Schelde" presently has 3,100 employees on its payroll. As of 1978, a total of 57 mesotheliomas had been diagnosed among them. Because of the long latent period for the development of mesothelioma, this type of cancer is expected to strike the Royal "de Schelde" workers for some time to come.

The menace turns up in France

Between 1956 and 1978, 70 cases of mesothelioma were observed in French shipyards in the region of Nantes and St. Nazaire, in Brittany. Extensive shipbuilding and ship repair was conducted in these yards following World War II. Since 1970, cases of mesothelioma have been increasing year by year among this workforce, and the disease is expected to occur among these men for many years to come. About 15,000 men worked in these shipyards in 1946; today the number is 10,000.

In most instances, the latent period for the development of mesothelioma among the French shipyard workers has proved to be more than 25 years. In one case, however, the latent period was only 11 years. This patient was first exposed to asbestos as a child, when his father, who was a shipyard lagger, is believed to have brought home asbestos dust on his work clothes.

Asbestos disease in U.S. shipyards

A health survey of 1,074 insulation workers in United States shipyards was conducted at the end of World War II. No significant evidence of disease was found upon X-ray examination of these workers, who, for the most part, had worked in the shipyards for 5 years or less. Unfortunately, it was not realized at the time that asbestosis and other asbestos-related diseases take at least 10 to 20 years to develop, and that X-ray evidence of disease could not be expected to occur until then.

During the 1960s, evidence that asbestos insulation workers in American shipyards were experiencing markedly increased death rates from cancer, mesothelioma, and asbestosis began to appear. However, workers in other trades in United States shipyards were not thought to be at risk until the terrible health effects of indirect exposure upon the British, Dutch, and French shipyard workers became known.

During 1975 and 1976, Dr. Selikoff and his colleagues at Mount Sinai conducted a clinical field survey of 1,000 shipyard workers at the General Dynamic Corporation's Electric Boat Division, in Groton, Connecticut. Groton is known as the submarine capital of the world. It is there that the first Nautilus and Trident nuclear submarines were built.

The health evaluation survey was requested by trade unions representing 14,000 of the 22,000 workers employed at the Groton shipyard. All of the 1,000 subjects in the survey were volunteers, and most had been employed there for 15–20 years or more. They included boilermakers, pipefitters, insulators, painters, carpenters, welders, electricians, machinists, laborers, office workers, draftsmen, and guards.

About half of these workers showed X-ray evidence of pulmonary and pleural abnormalities of the sort regularly seen in people who are occupationally exposed to asbestos dust. The abnormalities were found in all of the trades, indicating that conditions in the shipyard were such that asbestos exposure had occurred among all individuals working in the vicinity of asbestos operations.

Similar findings occurred in a health survey of 359 workers at two naval shipyards in the San Francisco Bay area. Moreover, X-ray examination revealed lung abnormalities in many workers at the Long Beach Naval Shipyard south of Los Angeles.

Since it is well known that asbestos exposure sufficient to cause mesothelioma can occur without showing up on X-rays, a grim question must now be posed. How many American shipyard workers will develop cancer and mesothelioma as a result of indirect occupational exposure?

Unfortunately, there is already some evidence that a terrible disaster may be in the making among the 3.5 million or so current and former shipyard workers of the nation. Epidemiologists from the National Cancer Institute, in Bethesda, Maryland, have recently discovered a significant excess of deaths from respiratory cancer among the residents of coastal Georgia, where two large shipyards were in operation during World War II, in Brunswick and Savannah.

What can be done about the shipyard environment?

In 1975, the use of asbestos in shipbuilding and ship repair was largely abandoned by the United States Navy and civilian yards. In spite of this belated action, ship repair still poses a thorny problem because asbestos previously used as insulation on steam pipes and boilers must be ripped out and replaced with nonasbestos materials during renovation and repair work. At the present time, there are 77 ship repair facilities in the United States under contract to the United States Maritime Administration. It is not clear what measures are being taken to prevent asbestos exposure in these facilities. Indeed, the United States Navy has been reluctant to allow Federal health agencies to inspect them. However, the following steps have been proposed to reduce dust levels in English shipyards:

- Limit the area of possible exposure by enclosing the work site.
- Suppress asbestos dust by wetting.

- Train personnel in careful work and clean-up procedures that will avoid the creation of dust.
- Provide suitable protective clothing and respirators.
- Use industrial vacuum cleaners to collect asbestos dust, and dispose of such material in a safe and proper manner.

What can be done for former shipyard workers?

At present there is no effective treatment for mesothelioma, and the outlook for patients with lung cancer is only somewhat better. However, other types of asbestos-related cancer, such as gastrointestinal cancer, can often be treated and cured if diagnosed soon enough.

Clearly, then, all current and former shipyard workers should be made aware of the fact that they are at risk of developing asbestos disease, and placed under strict medical surveillance. Since the risk of lung cancer and cancer of the esophagus is greatly multiplied by cigarette smoking, these workers should be thoroughly educated about the necessity to quit smoking. Workers and their physicians should also be made aware of any pulmonary X-ray changes. This is important in order to hasten treatment for respiratory infections that are known to trigger many deaths in persons suffering from asbestosis.

Chapter 8
Indirect Occupational Exposure

Perhaps the most ominous aspect of the asbestos disease now occurring in shipyard workers is the fact that the vast majority of the patients were not asbestos workers to begin with, and thus never handled asbestos directly. As we have seen, they were engaged in a great variety of trades and were exposed to asbestos as unsuspecting bystanders when products containing the mineral were applied to steam pipes, boilers, and bulkheads.

Unfortunately, many other groups of workers may also have sustained potentially dangerous indirect exposure to asbestos. The largest group consists of more than four million workers in the various building construction trades. It is estimated that 70 percent of the workers who have been exposed to asbestos are in this industry. These men include pipefitters, welders, electricians, plumbers, carpenters, and others who may have been on construction sites while fireproofing materials containing asbestos were sprayed on the structural steel of high-rise buildings, or other asbestos products were used.

Between 1958 and 1973, sprayed asbestos fireproofing materials were used in more than half of the large multi-story buildings constructed in the United States. Previously, asbestos spraying had been done since at least the early 1940s for acoustical or decorative purposes. In 1970, three million pounds of sprayed asbestos was used for fireproofing alone. Since it is estimated that about 25 percent of the sprayed fireproofing material failed to adhere to the structural steel, an enormous amount of asbestos was simply blown into the surrounding air.

Obviously, people working in the vicinity of such operations were indirectly exposed to asbestos. No one knows the extent of the health hazards these workers face. Nevertheless, a potentially serious risk can be inferred from the increasing numbers of mesotheliomas being reported in men and women who sustained indirect exposure to asbestos dust in shipyards during World War II.

In 1973, new EPA regulations effectively abolished the spraying of asbestos materials for fireproofing or decorative purposes.

Indirect exposure in the chemical industry

Between 1967 and 1971, 24 cases of mesothelioma were observed among workers at two chemical plants in Germany. Only 16 of the patients had sustained direct occupational exposure to asbestos. Nine of the victims had been indirectly exposed by working in areas where asbestos was being handled by others. Chest X-rays taken before the development of mesothelioma were available in 23 of the 24 cases. They showed that 17 patients had developed pleural thickening and pleural calcification.

In order to investigate the potential asbestos hazard among chemical workers, researchers from the Mount Sinai School of Medicine recently examined 185 maintenance workers at a large chemical plant in New Jersey. Chest X-rays showed that fully 38 percent of these workers had lung abnormalities consistent with asbestosis. Pleural thickening and calcification were found in a majority of this group.

Most of the men had never worked directly with asbestos, but had experienced indirect exposure by virtue of working in areas where asbestos was being used by others. The increased risk of lung cancer and mesothelioma among them remains to be studied.

Indirect exposure in electric power stations

As early as 1965, it was known that a potentially serious health problem existed among asbestos insulation workers employed at an electricity generating station in London. Ten years later, the tragic dimensions of the problem were defined in an official medical report. Among 77 insulation workers, there were 45 cases of asbestosis, including 13 cases of pleural calcification. Three of the men had developed lung cancer, and 8 had been struck down by mesothelioma.

Such a finding led to the conclusion that maintenance workers at other power stations might also be at risk from asbestos disease. A recent French study supports this theory. It shows that nearly half of a group of 55 power station maintenance workers have developed pleural thickening or pleural calcification.

Chapter 9

Asbestos and Cigarettes: a Deadly Combination

In their 1968 study of asbestos insulation workers in the New York–New Jersey metropolitan area, Dr. Selikoff and Dr. Hammond found an important co-carcinogenic effect between asbestos exposure and cigarette smoking. In fact, all 28 workers who died of lung cancer between 1963 and 1968 smoked cigarettes regularly. This suggested that asbestos workers who smoked were up to 90 times more likely to die of lung cancer than men who neither worked with asbestos nor smoked. Not surprisingly, Drs. Selikoff and Hammond recommended at the time that "asbestos workers who do not smoke should never start, and those now smoking should stop immediately."

During the past 10 years, there has been much new evidence to support this warning. For example, another study has shown that asbestos insulation workers who smoke are 8 times more likely to get lung cancer than those who do not smoke. Smoking also increases their risk of death from asbestosis and from cancer of the esophagus.

On the other hand, it appears that cigarette smoking has no effect upon the development of mesothelioma among asbestos insulation workers. Nor is there any apparent link between smoking and the risk of colon, rectal, or stomach cancer. Such findings contradict the theory put forth by some industry spokesmen that asbestos exposure without cigarette smoking is relatively harmless.

Striking confirmation that asbestos and tobacco forms a

deadly combination comes from the study of mortality among workers at the amosite asbestos factory in Paterson, New Jersey. Dr. Selikoff has found that lung cancer occurs approximately 6 times more frequently in these men than in cigarette smokers not occupationally exposed to asbestos dust. In addition, he reports that the lung cancer rate among them is about 90 times that of men who neither smoke nor work with asbestos.

Studies of Finnish miners and millers exposed to anthophyllite asbestos also indicate that asbestos and cigarette smoking combine to increase the risk of lung cancer.

Dr. Hammond and Dr. Selikoff now present new information indicating that asbestos workers who do not smoke have five times as much lung cancer as other nonsmokers. And when asbestos exposure increases the already very high lung-cancer risk of cigarette smokers five times, the result is catastrophic—one out of five deaths is due to lung cancer!

Thus, most occupational health experts agree upon the following admonition for anyone who is occupationally exposed to asbestos:

DON'T SMOKE!

Chapter 10
Caring for Sick Workers

As can be seen from the preceding chapters, the toll being taken by asbestos disease among the world's asbestos workers has become a human tragedy of immense proportions. Indeed, it has been estimated that 30 to 40 percent of all heavily exposed asbestos workers can be expected to die of cancer. Dr. Selikoff has projected that asbestos may be causing 10,000 cases of cancer a year in this country. Others have projected much higher levels—as many as 40,000 cases a year.

These grim predictions raise some profound social, political, and ethical questions. How is our society dealing with this occupational health diseaster? In short, how are we taking care of the diseased worker and his family?

Sad to say, the answer can be given in a single word.

Poorly.

Worker's compensation

In the ideal version of worker's compensation, the worker gives up his right to sue his employer for injuries suffered on the job. In return, state law gives him medical benefits and some weekly allowance without requiring him to prove fault on the part of the employer.

However, this ideal version of worker's compensation has rarely been realized. In fact, the present system of state compensation laws in this country has been a miserable failure. For example, in New York—a state with nearly 10 percent of the nation's population—only five persons a year receive compensation for cancer. One does not have to be much of a projectionist to realize that such a system is obviously inadequate to deal with the onslaught of industrial disease that the Department of Health, Education and Welfare has estimated to be killing 100,000 American workers each year.

Some people claim that worker's compensation laws have encouraged a form of "protected" murder. Others say that they reflect a sorry lack of will on the part of society to afford compassion and justice to the victims of occupational disease. Whatever the case, the situation is full of contradiction and irony. Consider the fact that during World War II many states in this nation did not even recognize the hazard of asbestosis, let alone give compensation to its victims. And not a single state gave compensation for asbestos-related cancer. Yet, during this same period, lung cancer connected with asbestos exposure was a compensable disease in Nazi Germany!

There are many reasons for the failure of worker's compensation in the United States. For one thing, it is largely based upon a system in which private insurance carriers sell insurance to employers at the lowest possible rates. Since increased employee claims cause increased insurance rates, these carriers have traditionally resisted granting benefits except those for clear-cut injuries or accidents. Until recent years, therefore, relatively few health compensation claims were processed. Even today the administrative procedures for proving job-related diseases are often unduly complex. Moreover, the burden of proof for asbestos disease is always placed on the worker, who must retain a lawyer and pay a high contingency fee if he hopes to succeed with his claim.

Industry discovered many years ago that the best way to keep compensation costs low was by making it hard for workers to win compensation claims. As a result, most serious workmen's compensation cases, such as those involving asbestos disease, are deliberately prolonged as much as two to three years from time of application. During this period, the income of the disabled worker often drops and his bills pile up. Many times he will die before the claim is upheld. By the use of such delaying tactics, an insurance carrier can often force him or his widow to sign a compromise agreement with greatly reduced benefits.

Over the years, industry has lobbied very successfully at the state level to limit compensation payments and impose statutes of limitation upon claims. Since legislators and working people have been generally unaware of the long latency periods involved in the development of such occupational diseases as asbestosis and asbestos-related cancer, statutes of limitation are common in the compensation laws of many states. As a result, unless a claim is made within a few years after the end of employment, eligibility for compensation is totally lost.

This means that by the time an asbestos worker develops lung cancer or mesothelioma, he is often ineligible for compensation.

Incredible as it may sound, two states (Louisiana and Mississippi) have yet to award anyone compensation for asbestosis. In some other states, the benefits are small enough to be ludicrous. Not long ago, a worker in Georgia who died of asbestosis incurred medical bills totalling more than $85,000. However, the state of Georgia had fixed a limit of $1,500 on medical costs for any one injury.

Workers have fared little better elsewhere in the United States. In Pennsylvania, for example, there are no provisions for partial disability from asbestos disease. And in New Jersey, the widow of a man who died of mesothelioma in 1975 was awarded $15 a week, an amount based upon the fact that when her husband had been employed by the Johns-Manville company back in the 1920s his wages were $17.75 a week.

It is obvious that the present fragmented system of worker's compensation is grossly inadequate and needs drastic overhauling. Some people have suggested that Congress enact a uniform national system of worker's compensation based upon the no-fault principle. Proponents of such legislation say that Federal compensation should include realistic payments for economic loss and full medical coverage. In addition, they urge that statutes of limitation be abolished.

Litigation

The failure of worker's compensation in America has given rise to an extraordinary number of lawsuits against the asbestos industry over the past 10 years. For example, Johns-Manville currently faces lawsuits involving asbestos disease which are estimated to total between $1.5 and $1.7 *billion!* Many of these lawsuits are third party actions. This is a proceeding against a party other than an employer in order to recover damages for injuries caused by exposure to asbestos in the workplace. These so-called third parties are usually asbestos producers and suppliers. They are being sued for product liability by asbestos workers who claim that they should have been warned about the health hazards associated with the use of asbestos.

Most of the damages won in third party lawsuits have been in the form of compensation for injuries actually suffered as a result of asbestos exposure. However, evidence has recently come to light indicating that many asbestos companies knew of the health hazards associated with asbestos more than 40 years ago, and deliberately undertook to conceal this knowledge from their workers and from the public. Because of such callous disregard for human health and life, punitive damages may now be awarded much more frequently in third party lawsuits involving asbestos.

Legislation has recently been introduced in Congress that will substantially relieve asbestos companies of pecuniary liability claims, and require the Federal government to pay them instead. It remains to be seen whether the American people will choose to assume that burden and to deprive diseased workers of the opportunity to bring third party actions against the asbestos industry.

A new role for physicians

Doctors in the United States have traditionally concentrated on treating illness, and have often resisted involvement in social problems. However, many people are now of the opinion that physicians should also be vitally concerned with the social and economic impact of occupational disease upon their patients.

Physicians, it is thought, should familiarize themselves with the worker's compensation laws in the states in which they practice. The physician can then advise a patient whose illness is related to his work about legal requirements for notification and statutes of limitation. If necessary, the doctor can direct his patient to an attorney or to a Legal Aid Society for further assistance. In this case, he should furnish an accompanying letter giving his diagnosis and opinion that the condition is work-related. Finally, physicians should be available to appear in court in support of any justifiable claim for occupational disease compensation.

The company physician

For many years, a company physician was considered immune from any legal action by a worker on the ground that there was no patient-doctor relationship. This is no longer the case. Under present law, a company physician becomes "at risk" the moment he has contact with a worker.

A recent lawsuit in California ended in a $300,000 verdict against a company physician who failed to inform a worker whom he had had X-rayed that the X-ray disclosed evidence of asbestosis.

As a result of such cases, industry is beginning to accept the concept that its medical employees are required to make appropriate disclosure of hazards and health conditions to employees and to the public at large. Failure to do so can now render them liable to criminal conviction with penalties ranging from the imposition of fines to imprisonment.

The role of society

Few people would disagree that society has an obvious responsibility to the half million American workers who are either being stricken with or dying of occupational disease each year. Indeed, the least we can do is make a greater effort to compensate our sick workers, insofar as it is possible to compensate them, for lost wages, lost health, and loss of dignity, not to mention their pain and suffering.

The sad fact is, however, that no amount of compensation can restore the health of a disabled asbestos worker, or ease the suffering of his family. In short, by definition, compensation always comes after the brutal reality of disease. It is, therefore, invariably a question of too little, too late.

Should we not then make every effort to prevent occupational disease from occurring in the future? After all, as one labor leader recently said, "It is not a requirement of the capitalistic system that a worker contribute his body and health to the gross national product."

Part III
PREVENTING OCCUPATIONAL ASBESTOS DISEASE

In the late 17th century, Bernardino Ramazzini, the father of occupational medicine, prowled ceaselessly through the workshops of Modena and Padua, observing the conditions in which tradesmen were toiling. It was Ramazzini's custom to go among the stonecutters, dye-house workers, and metal grinders, urging them to be aware of changes in wind direction, and always to work with their backs to the wind. Ramazzini realized that these artisans were dying of occupational disease because they were inhaling toxic substances. He understood the need for dust control and ventilation long before the invention of industrial exhaust machines. By warning workers to avoid exposure, he laid the foundation for preventive medicine and industrial hygiene.

In his *Treatise on the Diseases of Tradesmen,* Ramazzini urged his fellow physicians to care for workers. "Medicine, like jurisprudence," he declared, "should make a contribution to the well-being of workers and see to it that, so far as possible, they should exercise their callings without harm."

Ramazzini wrote this credo more than 275 years ago. If it had been adopted by the medical community and the rest of society at the start of the industrial revolution, the wretched situation of the asbestos worker might have been largely avoided.

Chapter 11

Methods of Control

Today, as far as is known, the complete prevention of asbestos disease could only be achieved if exposure to asbestos were reduced to zero. Unfortunately, it is not always possible to attain this ideal. Therefore, it is necessary to reduce exposure levels to as low as possible. There are several methods to reach this goal:

- Substitution of other materials for asbestos.
- Introduction of engineering controls and more efficient ventilation systems.
- Encouragement of better work practices.
- Enforcement of strict standards limiting the amount of asbestos dust concentrations in the workplace.

Substituting nonasbestos materials

In 1973, the EPA imposed a nationwide ban on the spraying of asbestos-containing fireproofing materials on the steel girders of high-rise buildings. Minerals such as rock wool, gypsum, and vermiculite were then substituted in this process. However, their long-term health effects remain to be studied. The same holds true for another asbestos substitute, attapulgate, a mineral whose small fibers may also be respirable.

Since the spraying of virtually any kind of fiber tends to contaminate the surrounding air, nonasbestos insulation products have been developed that can be applied to steel either by trowelling or by the use of adhesives. Nonasbestos insulation products are now widely used in shipbuilding and ship repair in many nations, including the United States and the Netherlands.

One of the leading substitutes for asbestos insulation is fiberglass, or fibrous glass. Although this material has been demonstrated to be carcinogenic when injected into the chest wall of test animals, it is suggested that it may not pose a hazard to humans because the individual fibers cannot be readily inhaled. Nevertheless, the safety of fiberglass and other mineral substitutes for asbestos is still under investigation.

Engineering controls and ventilation systems

Shortly after the Occupational Safety and Health Act took effect in 1971, the United States Department of Labor was pressured by organized labor into issuing a legally enforceable standard for exposure to asbestos dust. In order to comply with the new regulations, industry was forced to install new engineering controls and improved ventilation systems, and to alter many of its operating procedures. Occasionally, however, industry chose to shut down a factory rather than spend the money to clean it up. Here are two case studies:

Tyler, Texas

In the autumn of 1971, officials of the National Institute for Occupational Safety and Health (NIOSH) inspected the Pittsburgh Corning Corporation's asbestos insulation plant in Tyler, Texas. Thick layers of asbestos dust coated floors, ceilings, rafters, and other surfaces in the factory. Workers were using pitchforks to throw asbestos into feeding machines. Saws and scrap grinding machines lacked sufficient ventilation equipment. The dust collection system consisted of canvas bags beneath the roof, which were periodically emptied by machanical shaking, and gave off huge amounts of asbestos dust into the interior of the plant. Because of these conditions, some areas of the Tyler factory were too dusty to make accurate fiber counts. However, out of 138 air samples that were taken, 117 exceeded the standard of 5 fibers per cubic centimeter of air which was then in effect.

Following the NIOSH inspection, the Department of Labor's Occupational Safety and Health Administration (OSHA) gave Pittsburgh Corning until March 31, 1972 to complete extensive improvements in the ventilation and dust-control systems of the Tyler plant. Rather than comply, the company shut down the factory in February.

Today the health situation of the nearly 900 employees of this factory is being carefully monitored. The prognosis is not good. The Tyler plant was a sister factory of the notorious Paterson amosite insulation plant, and the Tyler employees will probably suffer much the same fate as their Paterson, New Jersey, counterparts.

Marshfield, South Carolina

In 1969, Raybestos Manhattan, Inc., acquired an asbestos textile factory in Marshfield, South Carolina. Conditions in this plant were extremely dusty. Asbestos fiber was fed into storage bins by pressurized lines that leaked. Fiber was removed from the bins by workers who pitchforked it into carts from which it was then hand fed into carding machines. Exhaust equipment for the carding machines was poorly designed and badly maintained. The spinning and twisting processes were dusty due to yarn breaks. Weaving was done dry and exhaust equipment on the automatic looms was inefficient.

Between 1969 and 1973, Raybestos Manhattan improved conditions in the Marshfield plant by redesigning and upgrading the carding machines and other dust-generating equipment, and by using wetted yarns in the weaving process.

Between 1973 and 1976, the company eliminated asbestos from products where a viable substitute could be found, and installed a $2.6 million "clean system" at the Marshfield plant for manufacturing products that contained asbestos. During this period, the entire carding process was enclosed and ventilated. Closed systems were also installed to eliminate the manual handling of asbestos fiber wherever possible. Fresh, clean air was provided to the workplace by new heated or humidified air units, and improved exhaust systems were installed in the spinning and twisting sections of the factory.

Operating and work practices

Since it was recognized that engineering alone could not maintain a sufficiently "clean" environment at the Marshfield plant, high priority was given by Raybestos Manhattan to the development of new work practices and administrative procedures. Here are some of them:

- Wetting down of asbestos waste before removal.
- Requiring personnel to wear protective clothing and respirators when entering enclosed areas to perform maintenance and clean-up.
- Continual use of industrial vacuum cleaners to remove waste.
- Patching tears and holes in all bags and packages containing raw asbestos fiber or finished goods in order to prevent the escape of airborne asbestos dust.
- Monitoring asbestos dust levels in all work areas to insure that workers are not exposed to excessive amounts of asbestos dust.
- Educating all employees about the necessity of maintaining a clean environment in the factory.

As a result of these improvements in engineering controls and work practices, Raybestos Manhattan says that all dust levels at the Marshfield plant are now well below the present Federal standard for exposure to asbestos, which is two fibers per cubic centimeter of air. The company claims that the Marshfield plant probably ranks as the cleanest factory of its kind in the world.

Other asbestos companies have also made tremendous improvements in dust control in order to come into compliance with Federal regulations. For example, most work stations in asbestos factories owned by the Johns-Manville Corporation are also well below the present Federal level.

This goes to show that in spite of its previous reluctance to spend money on dust control, the asbestos industry has the available technology to reduce asbestos exposure in a drastic manner. It means that we may be able to prevent asbestos disease from occurring in the future.

Sheldon W. Samuels, director of Health, Safety and Environmental Affairs for the AFL-CIO's Industrial Union Department, believes that such technology now makes it feasible for the Federal government to further lower the standard for occupational exposure to asbestos. "Standards can force the development of technology to protect the health of workers," he says.

Chapter 12

How Standards Are Set

The purpose of setting a standard or "threshold limit value" (TLV) for asbestos exposure is to prevent asbestos disease. TLV is a term meaning the highest level of a substance to which someone can be exposed without developing harmful effects. In order to set a meaningful TLV, it is essential to gather information on the dose-response relationship—the amount of asbestos exposure necessary to cause disease. Because of confusion and disagreement about the nature of this relationship, however, the setting of standards has always been a highly controversial matter.

Some scientists assume that there are levels of exposure to asbestos below which no adverse health effects will occur. Other scientists are dubious about this premise. They point to a recent monograph on asbestos published by the International Agency for Research on Cancer. It states that "at present, it is not possible to assess whether there is a level of exposure in humans below which an increased risk of cancer would not occur."

However, almost all of the medical experts agree that asbestos dust levels should be reduced as much as possible.

A history of asbestos standards

The first TLV for asbestos exposure was made by W. C. Dreessen and other scientists in the United States Public Health Service, in 1938, following a survey of nearly 500 employees in four North Carolina asbestos textile mills. Dreessen and his colleagues recommended a standard of 5 million particles per cubic foot of air for the prevention of asbestosis. At the time, they were unaware that inhalation of asbestos could cause cancer. But long after the carcinogenic effect of asbestos became known, the standard remained the same. In fact, the Dreessen standard survived as the only guide for controlling asbestos exposure in the United States for more than 30 years!

The 5 million particles in the Dreessen standard included asbestos fibers and all other airborne particles. This was a rather inaccurate way of measuring asbestos in a given volume of air, because the percentage of asbestos fiber in airborne dust could vary tremendously from plant to plant.

Another problem with the Dreessen guideline was that it was not enforceable by law. As a result, almost nobody bothered to abide by it. In 1960, the Dreessen TLV finally became legally enforceable under the Walsh-Healey Act, but only for those companies doing more than $10,000 worth of business with the Federal government.

In 1969, a Federal standard of 12 asbestos fibers longer than 5 microns per cubic centimeter of air was promulgated. This level was considered to be the equivalent of two million particles per cubic foot of air. The chief reason for counting fibers longer than 5 microns was that few laboratories were equipped with electron microscopes which are necessary to resolve the smaller particles. Since little or nothing was then known about the disease potential of fibers smaller than 5 microns, the new method of measuring asbestos lacked scientific foundation.

In December 1971, the 12-fiber standard was replaced by an emergency temporary standard of 5 fibers per cubic centimeter, and this was promulgated as a permanent standard in June, 1972. At that time, it was stipulated that by July 1, 1976, the 8-hour time-weighted average (TWA) of airborne concentrations of asbestos fiber to which any employee might be exposed should not exceed two fibers per cubic centimeter of air.

Is the two-fiber standard safe?

The two-fiber standard in effect in the United States today was first proposed by the British Occupational Hygiene Society in 1968. It was officially adopted in Britain in 1970. The standard was based on a study made in 1966 at an asbestos textile factory in Rochdale, England, which is owned by the Turner Brothers Asbestos Company, Ltd. This study suggested that a person working with chrysotile asbestos could be exposed for 50 years to a level of two fibers per cubic centimeter of air with only a 1 percent risk of developing asbestosis.

A more recent study of workers at the same factory, however, has raised considerable doubt about this prediction. The latest study suggests that between 7 and 24 percent of the workers might develop asbestosis after the 50-year period.

Even more alarming, a recent analysis of mortality among workers at this same factory suggests that approximately 3 percent of them might eventually die of asbestos-related disease, including cancer, following only 20 years of exposure to only one fiber per cubic centimeter.

The fact that the two-fiber asbestos standard now in effect in the United States and in England is designed only to prevent asbestosis and not cancer seems incredible in view of our knowledge that asbestos-related cancer is killing three to four times as many workers as asbestosis. At long last, however, government officials are finally beginning to recognize the necessity for lower levels of exposure to control lung cancer and other malignancies. Today, OSHA is proposing a new asbestos standard of 0.5 fibers per cubic centimeter of air. And NIOSH is recommending an ever lower level of 0.1 fibers per cubic centimeter.

The question is, which standard will be promulgated?

The asbestos standard debate

Because of recent doubt cast upon the validity of the two-fiber standard, there has been vigorous debate over just what level of exposure to asbestos should be set. Most industry spokesmen continue to state that the two-fiber standard is adequate to protect the health of asbestos workers. They point out that by today's standards many exposures in the past were incredibly high. They claim that the prevalence of disease among the asbestos insulation workers studied by Dr. Selikoff is a result of excessive exposure that no longer occurs. Industry representatives feel that a dose-response relationship has been established for asbestos disease and that lower exposure standards are unnecessary. They also emphasize that cessation of smoking by asbestos workers would reduce the risk of working with asbestos to what they call acceptable levels.

On the other hand, most trade union representatives, many members of the medical and scientific communities, and some government officials are doubtful that an acceptable standard for asbestos exposure can be established today. They point out that according to available scientific data it is not possible to predict a level of exposure to asbestos that will not result in the development of cancer, and that any level above zero entails some risk. They also believe that cigarette smoking should not be a consideration in the setting of asbestos standards since smoking has little or nothing to do with the development of mesothelioma or gastrointestinal cancer. Finally, they emphasize the fact that enforcement of asbestos standards has been flimsy at best, and that since OSHA has only 200 or so industrial hygienists to inspect 5 million workplaces, it is probably not going to improve.

The need for a new philosophy

The fact that the Federal standard for occupational exposure to asbestos has been reduced from 12 fibers to 5 fibers to 2 fibers per cubic centimeter of air over the past 10 years testifies to the government's inability to correctly assess the extent of the asbestos hazard. That further reductions in the allowable level of exposure appear imminent provides additional evidence of the consistent tendency on the part of the government to underestimate the problem and to settle for piecemeal solutions.

Short of an outright ban, then, how can we be sure that any new asbestos standard will be truly meaningful for the prevention of disease? Unfortunately, we cannot. Consider that the NIOSH proposal of 0.1 fibers longer than 5 microns per cubic centimeter means 100,000 of these long fibers in each cubic meter of air. Then consider that the average worker inhales about 8 cubic meters of air during a working day.

One great weakness of the various asbestos standards that have been issued over the years is that they invariably address the problem of preventing asbestos disease with technical jargon rather than in everyday language and in human terms. For example, a number of scientists have pointed out that the real problem is not fibers per thimbleful of air but *human lungfuls* of asbestos fiber. In this connection, Dr. Selikoff has said that an asbestos worker toiling in an environment that is supposed to contain two fibers longer than 5 microns per cubic centimeter of air may in fact be inhaling *800 million to 8 billion* asbestos fibers and fibrils of all sizes each working day.

To be sure, many of these inhaled particles may subsequently be exhaled, and thus expelled. On the other hand, as many as 50 percent may also be retained in the lungs of workers for whatever biological price they may eventually exact.

Should we not be thinking of the asbestos problem in terms of the human lung? And did Ramazzini not point the way toward such a philosophy 275 years ago when he urged tradesmen to work with their backs to the wind?

Part IV
THE ENVIRONMENTAL PROBLEM

Everyone appears to be surprised, these days, that we have an environmental problem with asbestos. They shouldn't be. Twenty years ago there was evidence that asbestos disease could strike well beyond the mine or the factory, endangering the health of workers' families and other residents of the community. The first clear warnings that asbestos could pose a serious environmental health hazard were sounded at the Conference on the Biological Effects of Asbestos, which The New York Academy of Sciences sponsored in 1964. Here are some of them:

- Dr. Raimo Kiviluoto told of finding calcification of the pleura in nearly 500 persons who had merely lived near anthophyllite asbestos mines in Finland. One 50-year-old woman had no known exposure to asbestos except that when she was 5 years old she lived for three months in the immediate vicinity of an asbestos mill, where she had sometimes played with bunches of asbestos fiber.
- Dr. J. C. Wagner told of finding mesotheliomas in South Africans who had not actually worked with asbestos, but merely lived in the vicinity of asbestos mines and mills. He described the case of a woman who had lived in a town in the asbestos fields until she was 5 years old. At the age of 55, she died of pleural mesothelioma. It turned out that as a child she was accustomed to slide down the side of an asbestos dump on her way home from school.

- Dr. Muriel L. Newhouse described cases of mesothelioma among relatives of asbestos workers, and among people living in the vicinity of an asbestos factory in London. A typical history of exposure was that of the wife who washed her husband's work clothes.
- Dr. J. G. Thomson told of finding evidence of inhaled asbestos fibers in the lungs of 25 percent of the people coming to autopsy at random in Cape Town, South Africa. Similar findings were reported from Miami and Pittsburgh.
- Dr. Wilhelm C. Hueper, of the National Cancer Institute, urged that the environmental health hazard posed by asbestos be thoroughly investigated. He advised the scientific community to determine the distribution pattern of asbestos. He said this should be done "from the site of its original occurrence and production through the sites and types of its subsequent industrial and commercial uses to the homes of the ultimate consumers."

Unfortunately, Dr. Hueper's sound advice went almost entirely unheeded. Massive amounts of asbestos continued to be sprayed on the steel girders of high-rise buildings throughout the United States. Asbestos was widely used in constructing the walls and ceilings of thousands of schools. Asbestos factories were allowed to exhaust air contaminated with asbestos fibers into the air of cities and towns across the nation. Asbestos workers were allowed to wear clothes contaminated with asbestos into their homes.

As for the consumer, asbestos found its way into practically every home in the land in a wide variety of products. It was used in wallboard and wallboard compound. It was an ingredient in pot holders and ironing board covers. It was a constituent in artificial embers, Christmas tree snow, and hair dryers. It was even used in papier-maché mixed by school children.

As a result of these miscellaneous uses and indiscriminate practices, asbestos has found its way into the lungs of an untold number of people in the general population, where it will remain for a lifetime. The following chapters describe what is known about the biological consequences of this, and some of the future problems that may now be anticipated.

Chapter 13
Unsuspecting Victims

As we shall see, asbestos disease can damage and destroy the health of people who are neither directly nor indirectly exposed to the mineral as a result of their work. Some of these unsuspecting victims have been the wives, children, and relatives of asbestos workers. Some have been residents of neighborhoods in which asbestos factories were located. Others are people who simply lived in the vicinity of shipyards where asbestos operations were conducted, or near asbestos mines and mills. And still others are exposed to harmful amounts of asbestos simply because they live in regions where asbestos deposits are located and where asbestos fibers can easily become airborne.

Within recent years, a number of studies have been made of the health experience of people who have been environmentally exposed to asbestos. Since their exposures have, for the most part, been far lower than those of the average asbestos insulation worker or factory worker, the discovery of disease and asbestos-associated abnormalities in them is highly disturbing.

It demonstrates once again that the disease-producing potential of the magic mineral has been seriously underestimated.

Family contact disease

The reader will remember that when investigators from the Mount Sinai School of Medicine studied the mortality experience of the 933 wartime workers at the amosite asbestos factory in Paterson, N.J., they found that more than half of the 200 excess deaths among these men were caused by cancer. They also found that 16 of the men had died of mesothelioma.

In recent years, a team of Mount Sinai researchers led by Dr. Henry A. Anderson, has studied the health experience of 679 household contacts of the 1,664 workers who were employed at the same factory between 1941, when it opened, and 1954, when it was shut down. The results of this study should be of grave concern to public health officials around the world.

None of these domestic contacts ever had personal occupational exposure to asbestos. None had ever set foot inside the Paterson factory. Yet fully 35 percent show asbestos-associated abnormalities when their lungs are X-rayed, as compared with only 5 percent in a control group.

Moreover, during the ongoing tracing of these people, whose only exposure to asbestos has come from merely living in the same household with a worker from the Paterson factory, 5 deaths have resulted from mesothelioma. The victims included:

- The 40-year-old son of a man who had worked in the factory for three years until the son was 11 years old.
- The daughter of the plant's chief engineer, who was 41 years old when she died.
- The 42-year-old daughter of a man who had worked in the plant for 5 years. When she was 10, she took lunch to her father at the plant every day. He met her at the doorway of the factory.
- A 32-year-old woman who at the age of 13 had lived in the home of her brother-in-law, a worker at the plant, for six months. Before that, she lived near the factory and often played in the homes of friends whose fathers worked there.
- The 50-year-old wife of an asbestos worker who had been employed at the plant for 8 years.

Since change rooms and company-laundered coveralls were not available at the Paterson factory, the source of home contamination is believed to have been asbestos dust adhering to the shoes, hair, and clothing of workers who returned home from the factory. However, the actual extent and intensity of this domestic exposure could only be estimated. In order to do this, each household contact was assumed to have had a duration of exposure equivalent to the length of time he or she lived in the same house with an asbestos worker.

As with many other studies of asbestos disease, the Paterson household investigation shows that increased duration of exposure, as well as increased time since first exposure, are associated with a higher rate of lung abnormality. For example, household contacts with more than 10 years of exposure had 4 times as much pleural thickening and 3 times as much pleural calcification as individuals with less than one year of exposure. As for increased time since initial exposure, 40 percent of the people first exposed between 1941 and 1946 had abnormal X-rays compared to only 22 percent for those who were first exposed between 1950 and 1954.

The Paterson household study clearly shows that under no circumstances should workers who are directly or indirectly exposed to asbestos bring their dusty clothes home to be laundered. Once asbestos gets into a home, it can remain for a very long time. Indeed, asbestos dust was found in the homes of former Paterson factory workers 20 years after the factory was shut down!

The Mount Sinai researchers are now undertaking to study the full extent of the disease risk that will be experienced by the household contacts of the Paterson workers. In the next few years, they hope to learn whether the relatively low levels of asbestos exposure experienced by this group will be sufficient to cause malignant disease other than mesothelioma.

Neighborhood exposure

Since the relatives of workers at the Paterson factory were known to be developing asbestos-associated abnormalities and disease through household exposure, the next step for the Mount Sinai investigators was to determine whether asbestos disease was occurring among people living in the vicinity of the plant. Dr. Hammond and Dr. Selikoff have explained their strategy as follows:

"We are studying defined populations that have been selected in terms of what appear to be diminishing levels of exposure to a known risk. Epidemiology is a bit like watching a rock thrown into a pond and measuring how far the ripples extend. In this case, of course, the rock is asbestos and the pond is the general community."

Dr. Hammond, Dr. Selikoff, and their colleagues had several reasons for thinking that people living in the neighborhood of the Paterson factory might be at some risk of developing asbestos disease. To begin with, mesothelioma had occurred among South Africans living near asbestos mines and mills, as well as among Londoners dwelling in the vicinity of an asbestos factory. Secondly, it was known that asbestos-contaminated air had been exhausted into the neighborhood of the Paterson plant. And, finally, the proprietor of a junk yard next to the Paterson factory had died of a pleural tumor in 1955.

In order to measure the effects a neighborhood exposure from the Paterson plant over a 35-year period, the Mount Sinai researchers traced 2,447 men who were living within one-half mile of the factory in 1942. (Men were chosen for the study because of the difficulty in tracing women whose names change with marriage and divorce.) The Mount Sinai investigators then determined the mortality experience of those men who died between 1962 (20 years after first exposure) and 1976. Finally, they compared this mortality exposure with that of several thousand men who had lived in 1942 in a neighborhood a few miles from the Paterson factory.

Happily, the results of the study so far do not indicate that the men who lived in the neighborhood of the Paterson factory have suffered any excess deaths from cancer or mesothelioma. (Indeed, their overall death rate from cancer is slightly lower than that of the control group.) However, since previous studies show that the latent period for the development of mesothelioma can be anywhere from 25–50 years, the Mount Sinai researchers plan to continue their investigation.

Asbestos air pollution

Since the Paterson factory was shut down in 1954, no one knows what levels of asbestos fiber may have contaminated the air of the surrounding neighborhood. However, there have been many surveys in recent years to measure asbestos levels in the urban environment. As a result, we know that asbestos fibers can be found in the air of practically any city in any industrialized country in the world.

Generally speaking, asbestos levels in the ambient air of European cities are between 0.1–10 nanograms per cubic meter of air. (A nanogram is one billionth of a gram.) Concentrations of asbestos in American cities have been somewhat higher, measuring anywhere between 0.1–100 nanograms per cubic meter of air. The highest concentrations have been found in New York City.

To be sure, these are extremely low levels compared with levels that have been measured in asbestos factories, mines, and mills. They are also far lower than the present Federal standard for occupational exposure to asbestos, which is the equivalent of between 10,000 and 100,000 nanograms per cubic meter. However, this does not mean that they should be dismissed as harmless. Asbestos levels ranging from 100–1000 nanograms per cubic meter have been measured in the homes of former asbestos workers. The highest level was below 5,000 nanograms. On the basis of the unfortunate health experiences of the household contacts of the Paterson workers, there is good reason to suspect that these low levels may have been sufficient to cause asbestos abnormalities and disease.

Another reason to worry about the amount of asbestos in the environment comes from France. Health officials of the French government have made extensive measurements of asbestos air pollution in the vicinity of a small plant in a heavily populated suburb of Paris in which asbestos sheets are cut. They have also measured asbestos levels one-half mile from a large asbestos factory in Normandy. In both places, they found asbestos levels ranging from 1000–3000 nanograms per cubic meter of air.

In urban areas not in the vicinity of asbestos factories, 99 percent of the measurements taken by the French investigators were below 7 nanograms per cubic meter, which is the level they consider to be an indication of asbestos air pollution.

No one knows for sure what asbestos levels existed during the 1960s in New York City and other American cities, where asbestos was routinely sprayed on the steel girders of high-rise buildings. Measurements taken by Dr. William J. Nicholson of the Mount Sinai School of Medicine indicate, however, that asbestos concentrations at rooftop level a quarter of a mile away from such spraying operations may have been as high as 1000 nanograms per cubic meter of air.

Whether mesotheliomas will develop in unsuspecting urban dwellers as a result of such exposures will not be known for at least another 10 to 15 years.

Chapter 14

A Turkish Nightmare

That asbestos could create a major public health problem in Turkey was first suggested in 1972. At that time, epidemiological studies revealed pleural calcification and pulmonary fibrosis in the lungs of people working in the asbestos mines of Anatolia, where there are large deposits of asbestos. Since then, the incidence of asbestos disease in Turkey has been studied extensively by Dr. Selahattin Yazicioglu and his co-workers at the Department of Chest Diseases of the Diyarbakir Medical Faculty, and by Dr. Y. Izzettin Bariş and some colleagues in the Chest Diseases Department of the Hacettepe University School of Medicine, in Ankara. They have discovered that environmental exposure to asbestos poses a major health hazard for many people in the general population.

Of even equal importance, perhaps, is that Dr. Bariş has found that pleural calcification, asbestosis, and malignant mesothelioma are endemic in certain villages of Turkey, where there are no asbestos mines, mills, or factories. Where, then, does the asbestos exposure come from? In some cases, it comes from rock outcroppings containing asbestos, which are common in those regions. The local residents have long been accustomed to use such rock for constructing their houses, and to plaster their homes with white stucco made from it.

Calcification of the pleura on X-ray examination has been found in many residents of these villages. Also, several hundred cases of mesothelioma have been reported among them, as well as a high incidence of lung cancer.

The curse of Karain

Karain is a village of about 600 inhabitants. It lies in the district of Ürgüp, which is well known to tourists because the people there live in picturesque rock dwellings called "fairy chimneys." Not so well known to the tourists is an old saying about the villagers of Karain. It goes as follows:

"First, the peasant of Karain falls ill with pain in the chest and belly. Then his shoulder drops and he dies."

Thanks to Dr. Bariş and his colleagues, it is now known what has been afflicting the peasants of Karain for all these years. It is mesothelioma, and they are dying of it at an unprecedented rate. Between 1970 and 1974, *half* the people who died in the village died of mesothelioma. In 1974, 11 out of the 18 deaths that occurred were due to this dread disease.

As of 1978, Dr. Bariş had verified 48 cases of mesothelioma in Karain. The average age at death was between 40 and 50. Some cases occurred in people who were in their thirties.

Since there were no asbestos deposits in the vicinity of Karain, however, Dr. Bariş was forced to look for another causative agent for mesothelioma.

As it happens, many fibers of respirable size can be found in samples of volcanic rock, road dust, and field soils taken in Karain. When examined under the electron microscope, these particles proved to be needle-shaped fibers of erionite. This is a type of zeolite—a large group of aluminum silicate minerals.

Dr. Bariş believes that zeolite fibers are the cause of the tragic death rate from mesothelioma in Karain, where the peasants build houses and dig cellars and storage caves out of the volcanic rock that is indigenous to the region.

High rates of pleural calcification, pulmonary fibrosis, and mesothelioma have also been seen in a number of other villages without natural asbestos deposits in the region of Karain. As a result, Dr. Bariş has suggested that all three diseases, which were formerly thought to be related only to asbestos exposure, can be caused by other fibers.

The fact that respirable erionite-type zeolite fibers appear to be the cause of mesothelioma and other lung disease is of considerable importance for other kinds of zeolites are important industrial materials. Because of their great capacity to absorb, zeolites are widely used in industrial filters. Zeolite is also used as a cracking catalyst in the manufacture of gasoline.

Needless to say, occupational exposure to zeolite fibers and other form of zeolite should now be carefully investigated, and appropriate preventive measures undertaken. There is already some reason to believe that a serious occupational problem may exist. Lung biopsies of two petroleum workers, who developed shortness of breath after being exposed to cracking catalysts, have shown the presence of zeolite particles. Health problems may also be posed by synthetic aluminum silicates, which are also being widely used in industry.

Because of Dr. Bariş, we have learned of still another cause of environmental lung disease. Experimental animal studies are now being conducted to determine the long-term pathological effect of zeolite fibers, as well as of other respirable fibers of similar structure.

Chapter 15

Contaminated Schools

Warnings were issued as early as 1971 that asbestos might pose a serious environmental hazard in school buildings across the nation. Asbestos pollution was found in a grade school in Wyoming, in a university dormitory in California, and in a library at Yale. In both the Wyoming school and the Yale library, asbestos concentrations were as high as 5 fibers per cubic centimeter of air—the Federal occupational standard at that time. In all three cases, public concern led to the removal of the asbestos materials that were causing the contamination. However, little was done to deal with the problem on a national level until 1977, when reports of asbestos exposure in New Jersey schools were widely published.

Today, the Environmental Protection Agency belatedly estimates that an asbestos hazard may exist in as many as 10,000 public schools in the United States. This astonishing and worrisome situation exists chiefly because asbestos was used extensively in school building construction between 1946 and 1973 as a component of fireproofing, insulation, and acoustical material.

Asbestos fibers are released from indoor materials such as ceiling and wall coatings through fallout and contact. Fallout of fibers comes from the aging and degradation of the bonding material in an asbestos-containing product. It is usually low level, continuous, and may increase with the age of the building.

Contact with asbestos-containing material, especially sprayed asbestos coatings, can easily result in the release of asbestos fibers. This is particularly true in school buildings, which tend to be subjected to extra wear and tear because of various student activities.

When fallen debris and dust containing asbestos particles are swept up by school maintenance workers, large amounts of respirable asbestos fibers can be resuspended in the air. Normal hustle and bustle by school children can have the same result. Once asbestos fibers become airborne in an indoor environment, they tend to stay aloft for long periods of time. In fact, some fibers can remain in the air—and, therefore, in the breathing zone of a person—for up to 80 hours.

Small wonder that high concentrations of airborne asbestos fibers have been measured in some of the nation's schools!

What is the government doing about this situation?

Incredible as it may seem, there are no Federal regulations governing indoor exposure to asbestos. Equally astonishing is the fact that the Clean Air Act of 1970 does not cover indoor pollution.

For some time, the EPA has been under pressure to promulgate rules for controlling the hazard under the Toxic Substances Control Act. However, although the Agency has funded research on fiber erosion from building insulation, it has not yet set standards or undertaken enforcement activity inside public buildings contaminated with asbestos.

While the government has been procrastinating, buildings grow older and more and more asbestos fibers are released. Dr. William J. Nicholson, of the Mount Sinai School of Medicine, has measured asbestos levels as high as 4,000 nanograms per cubic meter of air in Puerto Rican schools constructed of asbestos-cement material. And he has measured levels as high as 2,000 nanograms per cubic meter in public schools in the metropolitan New York area. Moreover, when Dr. Nicholson simulated the damage done by school children to ceilings containing asbestos, he obtained readings that were *nearly double* the present Federal standard for occupational exposure to asbestos.

In 1972, the National Cancer Institute reported that 12 cases of malignant mesothelioma had occurred in the United States between 1960 and 1968 in people under the age of 20. A recent case of mesothelioma in a school maintenance worker in Massachusetts has increased the suspicion among some researchers that asbestos pollution in the nation's schools may already be causing disease.

In Massachusetts, a special commission was created to investigate the asbestos hazard in schools. It found asbestos in student areas in 138 out of 1,200 schools that were surveyed. Widespread use of asbestos in schools has been reported in Indiana, Kentucky, and other states. If the estimates from the states already surveyed are applied to the entire nation, between 2 and 6 million students may be attending schools with asbestos surfaces in pupil areas. An additional 200,000 to 300,000 teachers could also be exposed.

Some states appear to be unconcerned about the asbestos problem in schools. Others have only minimal awareness of it. Approximately 260 New Jersey schools have been found to contain sprayed-on asbestos coatings. Forty-five of them had ceilings that were visibly flaking.

How can the problem be remedied?

Once observation or air sampling reveals the existence of an indoor asbestos hazard, there are two courses of action. The asbestos-containing material can be removed from the building. Or it can be encapsulated and contained through the use of a sealant.

Removal of asbestos material requires worker protection, environmental protection, and interruption of normal activities. Containment by encapsulation takes less time and is usually less expensive. However, encapsulation in school buildings should be limited to areas where contact damage will not occur. This precludes the use of sealants in many schools.

The cost of cleaning up the asbestos hazard in the nation's schools promises to be very high. For example, in 1976, in

Howell Township, New Jersey, flaking asbestos ceilings were removed from a school at a cost of $60,000. And in Newton, Massachusetts, $20,000 has been appropriated just to locate asbestos in one of the schools. Altogether, it is estimated that the total costs will run to literally hundreds of millions of dollars.

Some people are calling for Federal assistance to offset the costs of asbestos abatement programs in schools. Others say that the costs for detecting and remedying the hazard should be borne in part or in full by the manufacturers and distributors of asbestos-containing ceiling coatings.

During the past two years, the possibility that children, teachers, and maintenance workers are being exposed on a regular basis to hazardous concentrations of asbestos has evoked great concern in the United States. After much delay, the EPA is finally responding to this concern. During 1979, the agency has been lending technical help to the states for inspections of school buildings in which asbestos was sprayed on walls and ceilings. The agency says it is now preparing to require immediate action to reduce the asbestos hazard in schools that have not been examined or repaired under the technical assistance program. It is to be hoped that this will not turn out to be another case of too little, too late.

Meanwhile, of course, indoor asbestos pollution is not confined to 10,000 of the nation's schools. It is also a problem in thousands upon thousands of other structures in which asbestos spray operations were conducted, including office buildings, apartment dwellings, high-rise condominium complexes, libraries, and hospitals across the nation. Nor is the hazard confined to flaking walls and ceilings. It is also thought to exist in many air-conditioning systems that are contaminated with asbestos dust as a result of spraying operations that took place when these buildings were constructed. If this is the case, millions of unsuspecting Americans are being exposed to lower levels of asbestos air pollution.

Once again, the unanswered question is whether such lower level exposure will result in the development of mesothelioma 20 to 40 years from now.

Chapter 16
Future Environmental Problems

The fireproofing of structural steel in high-rise buildings goes back to the turn of the century. From then until shortly after World War II, fireproofing was accomplished by encasing the steel in layers of concrete. Following the war, the introduction of asbestos fiber sprayed-on coatings permitted equivalent fire protection with as little as one-fifth the weight of material and substantially less labor. Because of their exceptional fireproofing capabilities, asbestos coatings were also applied for decorative and acoustical purposes, including textural and soundproof ceilings.

As a result of this widespread use of sprayed-on asbestos materials, it is highly probable that asbestos coatings of some sort are present in almost any high-rise, steel-frame building constructed between 1946 and 1972. Just how much is not known. However, it has been estimated that during this period the average 30-story building was sprayed with 200 to 300 tons of fireproofing material. Other asbestos products can also be found in large buildings. These include pipe and boiler insulation, vinyl and asphalt asbestos floor tiles, and asbestos cement sheets.

As might be expected, asbestos pollution of the environment can occur when such buildings are demolished, remodelled, or repaired. As a result, the EPA has promulgated regulations dealing with the handling of asbestos materials during demolition and disposal, which are designed to avoid the creation of any health hazard. They include the following:

- Notification of the regional EPA office prior to demolition and disposal operations.
- Adequate wetting to prevent visible emissions during removal of asbestos material.
- Placing of asbestos material while still wet in leak-proof containers.
- Disposal of such material in designated areas.

In theory, the EPA regulations appear to promise effective control of asbestos demolition and removal operations. In reality, however, they are all too often neither obeyed nor enforced.

To begin with, contractors rarely bother to give notification. Secondly, so-called "adequate wetting" under the EPA rules can still result in dangerously heavy concentrations of asbestos. (For example, during a wet asbestos removal operation in one Massachusetts school, a level of *60 fibers per cubic centimeter* was measured!) In the third place, inadequate containers, broken bags, and disposal of dry asbestos are common. And, finally, asbestos waste is often disposed of as ordinary rubbish.

It seems obvious that asbestos contamination of the environment due to the demolition of buildings containing asbestos material continues to pose a threat to the public health. Stricter regulations may provide the answer to this problem. However, any and all regulations governing the handling of asbestos material will have to be rigorously enforced by Federal, state, and local authorities if the present situation is to be remedied.

Asbestos and drinking water

Pollution of public drinking water supplies in the United States is widespread. Indeed, there are almost daily reports of such occurrences. Usually the contamination is caused by chemical agents, but drinking water pollution can also be caused by mineral fibers.

In Silver Bay, a town on Lake Superior in eastern Minnesota, taconite ore mined in the Mesabi Range is processed and iron is extracted. The leftover tailings are then dumped as a slurry into a man-made delta in the lake. Since about 1961, it is estimated that 67,000 tons of taconite tailings a day have been disposed of in this manner.

In 1972, it was discovered that 20 percent of the taconite ore from the Mesabi Range contained an asbestos-type mineral. It was also discovered that mineral fibers similar to (and in some instances indistinguishable from) amosite asbestos were contaminating the drinking water supplies drawn from Lake Superior by Duluth, a city of 100,000 inhabitants located 50 miles from Silver Bay.

Dr. Arthur M. Langer, a mineralogist at the Mount Sinai School of Medicine, has identified the mineral fibers in Duluth drinking water as grunerite. (Asbestiform grunerite is commonly known as amosite asbestos.) Whether or not these grunerite fibers will pose a health hazard to the residents of Duluth and to other people drinking water from Lake Superior is unknown at the present time.

The current OSHA threshold limit value of two fibers per cubic centimeter of air translates roughly into an exposure of between 10 and 15 million fibers per working day. Some researchers estimate that about one-half of all inhaled asbestos fibers will enter the gastrointestinal tract, and they assume that this is the reason for the increased rate of gastrointestinal cancer among asbestos workers.

For his part, Dr. Langer has estimated that someone drinking a liter of Duluth water a day could be ingesting several million mineral fibers of a type similar in structure to amosite asbestos. He points out that the broad relationship between grunerite fiber and amosite asbestos provides good reason for public health concern about the situation in Duluth. He is especially concerned because of the excess kidney cancer and gastrointestinal cancer found in workers at the Paterson amosite asbestos factory.

What should be done about the situation in Duluth? Industry claims that there is no evidence that the mineral fibers in the drinking water there pose any health hazard whatsoever. But John P. Hill, who represented the Department of Justice before the Federal court in Minnesota, has another view:

"We know asbestos is in the drinking water," he says. "We know that when ingested it traverses the human system and is expelled through the bladder. And we know asbestos is a human carcinogen. Those of us with no economic interest to protect know it should be removed from the water. To do this, the uses of asbestos which caused it to be in the drinking water should be stopped."

Asbestos in strange places

Who would have thought that asbestos was being used in the manufacture of hair dryers? Or in artificial ashes, embers, and Christmas tree snow? Or, for that matter, as a dry ingredient in papier-maché mixed by school children in New York City schools?

The fact is that asbestos was not only used in all these products, but also without any label whatsoever warning of its presence!

The Consumer Product Safety Commission has recently banned the "intentional addition" of asbestos in artificial embers and ashes as well as in patching compounds that are widely used in wall repair and home remodelling. This, however, is just a drop in the bucket. According to the Commission, several thousand consumer products contain asbestos. Moreover, the regulation regarding "intentional addition" is extremely weak. Further, since there is no reliable method of determining if a product is releasing asbestos fibers, how can a manufacturer—or, for that matter the Commission—know if contamination is occurring? How then can the Commission enforce its own regulation? It is a classic *Catch-22* situation.

One answer to the dilemma would be to remove all items containing asbestos from the marketplace. However, this could prove economically disruptive. It might also result in the widespread use of asbestos substitutes that have not been tested for their long-term health effects. Another solution might be to require manufacturers to state on the label that their products *do not* contain asbestos. This is presently happening with many wall compounds that formerly contained the mineral.

Today there is little effort on the part of the government to determine which end products contain asbestos. The consumer is thus kept in the dark. And when asbestos or some other toxic agent is discovered in a household product, he is often as not bewildered by a spate of denials and conflicting viewpoints concerning the hazard involved.

Perhaps the best interim advice in this matter has been given by Dr. Selikoff, who says that "wherever you can identify something that has free-floating asbestos in it, keep it away from your children."

Clearly, a national policy for tracing and governing the use of asbestos in consumer products is in order if environmental pollution is to be avoided and the public health protected. It is interesting to note that if the country had followed the advice of Dr. Wilhelm C. Hueper, of the National Cancer Institute, such a program could have been started 15 years ago.

Part V
PUBLIC CONTROL OF ASBESTOS DISEASE

We are a nation in which between 8 and 11 million men and women have been exposed to asbestos in their work, and are officially recognized to be at risk of developing asbestos disease.

We are a nation with untold numbers of people in the general population who have been exposed to low-levels of respirable asbestos materials sprayed on steel girders during the construction of high-rise buildings, and who continue to be exposed to asbestos fibers as a result of living and working in those buildings.

We are a nation in which as many as 10,000 schools are estimated to contain asbestos surfaces that can give off potentially hazardous levels of asbestos into air breathed every day by millions of school children and by several hundred thousand teachers.

We are, therefore, a nation that is already afflicted by an occupational health disaster for its asbestos workers, and one that could be subjected to an environmental health disaster among people in the general population.

In short, we are a nation with a national asbestos public health problem.

What can we do about it? How can we go about implementing public health control of occupational and environmental asbestos disease? Which segments of society are responsible for taking the kind of preventive measures today which will insure the public health tomorrow? Who is making himself heard on this issue? And what are some of the stumbling blocks?

The following chapters will attempt to answer some of these questions.

Chapter 17
What Should Society Be Doing?

The best method for society to control the massive problem of asbestos disease that confronts the nation is through governmental regulation. The government's role is obviously to protect all citizens—be they workers or members of the general population—from any exposure to asbestos that will result in disease. The most effective way for the government to go about this is to control asbestos dust emissions at their source. But in order to do that, the government must promulgate and enforce asbestos emission standards that are low enough to prevent asbestos disease from occurring.

As things stand, OSHA's present occupational standard for asbestos exposure does not fulfill this basic requirement. It is designed merely in the hope that it will prevent asbestosis, or lung scarring. The deficiency of such a standard is evident in the fact that for the past 10 or 15 years almost every study of death among asbestos workers shows that the great majority of them are dying of cancer, not asbestosis. Most researchers believe that cancer can be caused by levels of asbestos exposure far lower than those necessary for the development of asbestosis. And most occupational cancer experts believe that there is *no* safe level of exposure to a cancer-causing substance.

As for the EPA, its present standard for protecting the public against environmental exposure to asbestos merely states that there shall be no *visible* emissions of asbestos. .This, of course, is absurd since most asbestos fibers are invisible to the naked eye. Indeed, asbestos fiber counts in invisible emissions can exceed 10 fibers per cubic centimeter of air. This level is 5 times greater than the 8-hour time-weighted average of airborne concentrations of asbestos fiber presently in effect for occupational exposure. One of the chief reasons for the EPA's sorry record regarding asbestos exposure is that the agency does not have the necessary equipment to measure such levels of exposure.

What can be done to remedy this incredible situation in which neither workers nor people in the general population are being afforded sufficient protection against asbestos disease?

- OSHA should promulgate without delay a standard that will protect all workers—including workers indirectly exposed to asbestos—from the risk of developing asbestos-related cancer. Since the dose-response relationship (i.e., the amount of asbestos exposure necessary for the development of cancer) remains unknown, such a standard must include a large built-in margin of safety. In other words, it should eventually be as close to zero as possible. The least OSHA should do as a starter is to promulgate the 0.1 fibers-per-cubic-centimeter standard proposed by the National Institute for Occupational Safety and Health. Only in this way can an end be put to the trial-and-error method of standards-setting that has, in effect, used workers as test animals in determining the long-term disease producing potential of asbestos.
- The EPA should promulgate and rigorously enforce indoor and outdoor emission standards for asbestos that will also contain a large built-in safety margin for the prevention of cancer. (The fact that it is now perfectly legal for people in the general population to be exposed at home and at work to the same levels of asbestos mandated for factory workers is intolerable.) Needless to say, the EPA should be given the proper measuring equipment to perform this task. The fact that asbestos exposure of low but widely varying degree is occurring in thousands of schools, office buildings, and apartment dwellings makes this action a national health priority of the utmost importance.
- The Consumer Product Safety Commission should ban all products from the marketplace that give off free-floating asbestos fibers when used or installed by consumers.

In short, governmental policy toward public control of asbestos disease should at long last be geared to the concept of *prevention.*

The role of industry

The goal of industry must be the responsible use of asbestos. This requires ongoing surveillance of asbestos from the time it is mined and milled, through the process of using it in the manufacture of various products, until it is purchased and used by the consumer. In short, the producers of asbestos must concern themselves with users and end users of their asbestos products.

Dr. Paul Kotin, medical director of the Johns-Manville Corporation, the world's leading producer of asbestos, has defined this responsibility as follows:

"It has become and will continue to become advisable to discontinue selling asbestos fibers in several markets where the end product does not lock in the fibers to reduce to the ultimate the possibility of those fibers become airborne," he says. Dr. Kotin believes the same policy should hold true when it is impractical to control the end uses of a product in a way that will avoid creating respirable asbestos dust. "In a word, the producer and the manufacturer has the responsibility for educating the user of the product and limiting the use of the product to acceptable and nonhazardous uses," he declares.

Organized labor—a watch dog

It goes without saying that a basic policy of any trade union should be to protect the health of its members as well as their economic interest. This is why many labor leaders have taken a strong stand on the problem of asbestos exposure. Charles Levinson, director of the International Federation of Chemical, Energy, and General Workers' Unions, has called for the formation of health registers for all people exposed to asbestos in order to facilitate medical follow-up. "The only responsible and reasonable definition of safety can be no exposure or the lowest possible level of exposure," he says.

Sheldon W. Samuels, of the AFL-CIO's Industrial Union

Department, points out that OSHA's proposed asbestos standard of 0.5 fibers per cubic centimeter of air is based only on feasibility. "There has never been a workplace or community environmental standard that was based solely on biological data," he declares. Samuels claims that the new asbestos standard should not be based upon the best *available* technology but upon the best *possible* technology. For this reason, he favors the NIOSH proposal of 0.1 fibers per cubic centimeter of air.

Like many labor leaders, Samuels is scornful of industry's espousal of the concept of "acceptable risk." Samuels says this is "like playing Monopoly with the Mafia, who always start the game owning the Boardwalk." He points out that the reduction of risk in the workplace is a 100-year-old struggle in the United States. "There never was any historical or social 'acceptability' of risk," he declares.

Roy J. Steinfurth, of the International Association of Heat and Frost Insulators and Asbestos Workers, says that organized labor will no longer accept scientific conclusions reached by industry-controlled scientists. "The crimes that have been committed in the past must cease and be paid for," he has said. "The withholding of information pertaining to all occupational disease, not just asbestos-related disease, should be made a criminal offense and punishment dispensed accordingly."

The role of law

We are a nation living under laws that are designed to protect the lives and rights of our citizens. Yet our laws governing occupational exposure to asbestos have failed to prevent wholesale disease and death from occurring among the asbestos workers of America. Our fragmented system of state-by-state worker's compensation laws has failed miserably to ease the economic burden of the sick worker and his family. Liability lawsuits against industry are settled on a costly and time-consuming case-by-case basis, so they have not been an effective means of dispensing justice either.

A highly controversial bill has been introduced in Congress to remedy this situation. Entitled the *Asbestos Health Hazards Compensation Act,* it would eliminate further product liability or third party actions against the asbestos industry. It would use the Federal treasury to pay off existing claims for liability, and then set up an industry fund to pay compensation to anyone developing asbestos disease in the future.

Proponents of this bill argue that it would dispense relief to afflicted asbestos workers on an impartial basis. They point out the indisputable fact that for many sick asbestos workers and their families, the future is terribly bleak unless some kind of aid is forthcoming.

Critics of the measure point out that it was drafted by lawyers connected with the asbestos industry, and claim that it was primarily designed to benefit industry rather than the victims of asbestos disease. They say that the burden of proof to show disability will still fall unfairly upon the worker.

According to the proposal, the reason for relieving asbestos companies of financial liability is that "the scope of diseases causally related to asbestos and/or cigarette tobacco smoke was unknown to industry, labor, government, or medicine until recent times."

Karl Asch, a leading New Jersey attorney in asbestos litigation, scoffs at this contention, pointing out that the dangers of asbestos inhalation were recognized in Anglo-American jurisdictions as far back as 1931. Asch also points to the recent discovery that the asbestos industry in the United States suppressed evidence about asbestos disease way back in the early 1930s.

"It is difficult to understand why the American taxpayer should pick up the costs for those who sowed the seeds of asbestos death and disease," he says.

Meanwhile, as the issue is argued back and forth, the laws of our land remain inadequate for protecting the health of asbestos workers, and for compensating them when they fall sick with asbestos disease.

Chapter 18
The Lesson of Asbestos Disease

What can the average citizen learn from the tragedy that has overtaken the asbestos workers of the world? Here are a few things to remember:

- The human lung is a delicate and fragile mechanism. It was not intended to serve as an industrial vacuum cleaner. Nor was it intended to filter out asbestos particles from the air of our cities and school rooms. Indeed, the human lung should never undergo any unnecessary exposure to asbestos dust.

- A nation that cannot summon the will to protect the lungs and the health of its workers cannot very well protect the lungs and the health of the rest of its citizens. The reason is absurdly simple: workers make products that are used by everyone else. Asbestos is a perfect example. After all, if we had been willing to recognize that asbestos was a hazard for our workers, would we have allowed it to contaminate the classrooms of our schools?

- Asbestos disease, like most other occupational diseases, does not strike down its victims quickly. It works slowly and insidiously over a long period of time. Indeed, one day of exposure is considered by some scientists to be sufficient to cause fatal cancer two decades later. In a sense, asbestos is an invisible bullet that takes 20 to 40 years to kill. Therefore, preventive measures against future asbestos disease must be taken *now*.

In 1973, Dr. Selikoff put the problem to the United States Senate Commerce Committee as follows:

"Prevention of cancers in the year 2,000 has to be our concern in 1973," he said. "It is what is happening in 1973 which will become evident in the year 2000."

It is now 1980.

What are we doing to prevent asbestos disease today?